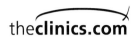

CLINICS IN GERIATRIC MEDICINE

Diabetes

GUEST EDITOR
John E. Morley, MB, BCh

August 2008 • Volume 24 • Number 3

SAUNDERS

An Imprint of Elsevier, Inc.
PHILADELPHIA   LONDON   TORONTO   MONTREAL   SYDNEY   TOKYO

W.B. SAUNDERS COMPANY
A Division of Elsevier Inc.

1600 John F. Kennedy Blvd., Suite 1800 • Philadelphia, PA 19103-2899

http://www.theclinics.com

CLINICS IN GERIATRIC MEDICINE
August 2008
Editor: Lisa Richman

Volume 24, Number 3
ISSN 0749-0690
ISBN-13: 978-1-4160-6301-8
ISBN-10: 1-4160-6301-3

Clinics in Geriatric Medicine (ISSN 0749-0690) is published quarterly by Elsevier Inc., 360 Park Avenue South, New York, NY 10010-1710. Months of issue are February, May, August, and November. Business and Editorial Offices: 1600 John F. Kennedy Blvd., Suite 1800, Philadelphia, PA 191023-2899. Customer Service Office: 6277 Sea Harbor Drive, Orlando, FL 32887-4800. Periodicals postage paid at New York, NY, and additional mailing offices. Subscription prices is $189.00 per year (US individuals), $327.00 per year (US institutions), $246.00 per year (Canadian individuals), $398.00 per year (Canadian institutions), $246.00 per year (foreign individuals) and $398.00 per year (foreign institutions). Foreign air speed delivery is included in all *Clinics* subscription prices. All prices are subject to change without notice. POSTMASTER: Send address changes to *Clinics in Geriatric Medicine*, Elsevier Periodicals Customer Service, 6277 Sea Harbor Drive, Orlando, FL 32887-4800. **Customer Service: 1-800-654-2452 (US). From outside of the United States, call 1-407-563-6020. Fax: 1-407-363-9661. E-mail: JournalsCustomerService-usa@elsevier.com.**

Reprints. For copies of 100 or more of articles in this publication, please contact the Commercial Reprints Department, Elsevier Inc., 360 Park Avenue South, New York, New York 10010-1710 Tel.: (212) 633-3812; Fax: (212) 462-1935, E-mail: reprints@elsevier.com.

Clinics in Geriatric Medicine is covered in *MEDLINE/PubMed (Index Medicus), EMBASE/Excerpta Medica, Current Contents/Clinical Medicine (CC/CM), and the Cumulative Index to Nursing & Allied Health Literature.*

Printed in the United States of America.

GUEST EDITOR

JOHN E. MORLEY, MB, BCh, Geriatric Research Education and Clinical Center, St. Louis VA Medical Center; and Geriatric Medicine, Saint Louis University School of Medicine, St. Louis, Missouri

CONTRIBUTORS

STEWART G. ALBERT, MD, Professor of Internal Medicine, Department of Internal Medicine, Division of Endocrinology, Saint Louis University School of Medicine, St. Louis, Missouri

WILBERT S. ARONOW, MD, Clinical Professor of Medicine, Divisions of Cardiology, Geriatrics, and Pulmonary/Critical Care; Chief, Cardiology Clinic; and Senior Associate Program Director and Research Mentor for Fellowship Programs, Department of Medicine, Westchester Medical Center/New York Medical College, Valhalla, New York

NICOLE DUCHARME, DO, Division of Endocrinology, Saint Louis University Medical Center, St. Louis, Missouri

KENNETH PATRICK L. LIGARAY, MD, Instructor of Medicine, UAB Health Center Montgomery, University of Alabama School of Medicine, Montgomery, Alabama

ANGELA D. MAZZA, DO, Fellow, Division of Endocrinology, Saint Louis University, St. Louis, Missouri

JOHN E. MORLEY, MB, BCh, Geriatric Research Education and Clinical Center, St. Louis VA Medical Center; and Geriatric Medicine, Saint Louis University School of Medicine, St. Louis, Missouri

ABHIJEET A. NAKAVE, MBBS, Research Fellow, Strelitz Diabetes Institutes, Department of Internal Medicine, Eastern Virginia Medical School, Norfolk, Virginia

CHHAYA V. PATEL, MBBS, Research Fellow, Strelitz Diabetes Institutes, Department of Internal Medicine, Eastern Virginia Medical School, Norfolk, Virginia

E. SHARON PLUMMER, RN, BC, GNP, Gerontological Nurse Practitioner and Certified Diabetes Educator, Department of Internal Medicine, Division of Endocrinology, Saint Louis University School of Medicine, St. Louis, Missouri

RANI RADHAMMA, MD, Division of Endocrinology, Saint Louis University Medical Center, St. Louis, Missouri

NEELAVATHI SENKOTTAIYAN, MD, Division of Endocrinology, Saint Louis University Medical Center, St. Louis, Missouri

ALAN B. SILVERBERG, MD, FACP, FACE, Professor of Internal Medicine, Division of Endocrinology, Department of Internal Medicine, St. Louis University School of Medicine, St. Louis, Missouri

ELSA S. STROTMEYER, PhD, MPH, Assistant Professor, Center for Aging and Population Health, Department of Epidemiology, Graduate School of Public Health, University of Pittsburgh, Pittsburgh, Pennsylvania

DAVID R. THOMAS, MD, FACP, Professor of Medicine, Division of Geriatric Medicine, Saint Louis University Health Sciences Center, St. Louis, Missouri

NINA TUMOSA, PhD, Associate Director for Education, Geriatrics Research, Education, and Clinical Center, St. Louis Veterans Administration; and Professor of Internal Medicine, Division of Geriatrics, Saint Louis University, St. Louis Veterans Administration Medical Center, St. Louis, Missouri

AARON I. VINIK, MD, PhD, Strelitz Diabetes Institutes, Department of Internal Medicine, Eastern Virginia Medical School, Norfolk, Virginia

CONTENTS

stroke, peripheral arterial disease, and of congestive heart failure. This article reviews studies addressing the implications of hypertension and the older diabetic.

Diabetes mellitus is among the most common and complex chronic diseases that affect approximately 20 million individuals in the United States. An additional 26% of the population has impaired fasting glucose, making diabetes an epidemic. MNT in diabetes addresses not only glycemic control but also other aspects of metabolic status, including hypertension and dyslipidemia, which are major risk factors for cardiovascular disease. MNT is an integral component of diabetes management, which includes the process and system through which nutritional care and specific life style recommendations are provided to diabetic individuals. Cultural and ethnic preferences are taken into account and patients are involved in the decision-making process.

Elderly diabetic persons are 1.5 times more likely than age-matched nondiabetic persons to develop vision loss and blindness. Annually, between 12,000 and 24,000 diabetic patients in the United States become legally blind because of complications caused by diabetic retinopathy. Even more diabetic persons experience vision loss caused by comorbid ocular and periocular conditions such as dry eye syndrome, cataracts, macular degeneration, and glaucoma. This article discusses the synergy between these conditions and diabetes. Standards of care that slow the progression of vision loss and exciting new research on new strategies of care that may reverse vision loss are presented.

Anemia is common in diabetic patients and is associated with increased morbidity and mortality. The observations that diabetes-related chronic kidney disease is more common than chronic kidney disease of other etiologies, that anemia may occur earlier in diabetes-related chronic kidney disease than in other types of chronic kidney disease, and that anemia in diabetes-related kidney disease often is found without measurable renal impairment suggest that the diabetic population may have a predilection to the development of anemia. Anemia is associated with a poorer prognosis in diabetic-associated comorbid conditions, but targeted correction of anemia has improved diabetic patients' quality of life.

FORTHCOMING ISSUE

November 2008
Perioperative Management
Amir Jaffer, MD, *Guest Editor*

THE CLINICS ARE NOW AVAILABLE ONLINE!

Access your subscription at:
www.theclinics.com

ELSEVIER
SAUNDERS

Clin Geriatr Med 24 (2008) xi–xiii

CLINICS IN
GERIATRIC
MEDICINE

Preface

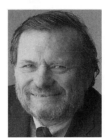

John E. Morley, MB, BCh
Guest Editor

*Life is not over because you have diabetes. Make the most of what you have,
be grateful.*

—Dale Evans Rogers

The last issue of *Clinics in Geriatric Medicine* on diabetes mellitus was published nearly 10 years ago [1]. In the last 10 years there have been dramatic advances in our understanding of diabetes and its treatment. There has been an exponential increase in articles on diabetes mellitus in the elderly [2,3]. Diabetes occurs in nearly 20% of people older than 65 years of age and insulin resistance occurs in half of older individuals [4,5]. Diabetes is now recognized to cause sarcopenia, frailty, falls, and hip fractures [6–8]. These issues, along with the dramatic advances in the diagnosis and treatment of diabetic neuropathy, are discussed in the first articles.

Thomas Willis in the 18th century suggested that "Diabetes is caused by melancholy [9]." In the last decade there has been increasing awareness of the effects of depression and cognitive dysfunction on the ability of individuals to control their diabetes [10,11]. The role of HbA$_1$C monitoring in nursing homes has been questioned [12,13]. The importance of managing lipids and blood pressure along with blood glucose has become more emphasized [14–16]. This emphasis has increased the problem of polypharmacy in older people who have diabetes [17]. All these concerns are discussed in detail in this issue.

0749-0690/08/$ - see front matter. Published by Elsevier Inc.
doi:10.1016/j.cger.2008.04.001

geriatric.theclinics.com

Finally, there has been an explosion of new therapies for diabetes mellitus over the last 10 years [18,19]. The use of these new therapies has to be balanced against their potential ill effects, as was demonstrated with the negative cardiovascular effects of rosiglitazone [20]. The difficulties in how aggressively to control diabetes in older people were highlighted by the early stoppage of the Action to Control Cardiovascular Risk in Diabetes (ACCORD) trial because of increased cardiovascular mortality. The role of medical nutrition therapy in older people remains controversial with questions concerning the potential negative consequences of weight loss [21] and the role of therapeutic diets [22].

This issue highlights the complexities of diabetes in older people and the difficulties and uncertainties in its management. When Nell Carter was first diagnosed with diabetes she denied it. It is clear that the one thing that neither the patient nor the physician can afford to do is to ignore diabetes.

John E. Morley, MB, BCh
Geriatric Medicine
Saint Louis University School of Medicine
1402 South Grand Boulevard
M238, St. Louis, MO 63104, USA

E-mail address: morley@slu.edu

References

[1] Morley JE. An overview of diabetes mellitus in older persons. Clin Geriatr Med 1999;15(2): 211–24.

[2] Kim MJ, Rolland Y, Cepeda O, et al. Diabetes mellitus in older men. Aging Male 2006;9(3): 139–47.

[3] Mazza AD, Morley JE. Update on diabetes in the elderly and the application of current therapeutics. J Am Med Dir Assoc 2007;8(8):489–92.

[4] Morley JE. Diabetes mellitus: A major disease in older persons. J Gerontol A Biol Sci Med Sci 2000;55(5):M255–6.

[5] Banks WA, Willoughby LM, Thomas DR, et al. Insulin resistance syndrome in the elderly: assessment of functional, biochemical, metabolic, and inflammatory status. Diabetes Care 2007;30(9):2369–73.

[6] Morley JE. Is weight loss harmful to older men? Aging Male 2006;9(3):135–7.

[7] Morley JE, Kim MJ, Haren MT, et al. Frailty and the aging male. Aging Male 2005;8(3–4): 135–40.

[8] Miller DK, Lui LY, Perry HM 3rd, et al. Reported and measured physical functioning in older inner-city diabetic African Americans. J Gerontol A Biol Sci Med Sci 1999;54(5): M230–6.

[9] Available at: http://en.thinkexist.com/quotes/Dale_Evans_Rogers/. Accessed April 17, 2008.

[10] Messinger-Rapport BJ, Morley JE, Thomas DR, et al. Intensive session: new approaches to medical issues in long-term care. J Am Med Dir Assoc 2007;8(7):421–33.

[11] Strachan MW, Price JF, Frier BM. Diabetes, cognitive impairment, and dementia. British Med J 2008;336(7534):6.

[12] Meyers RM, Broton JC, Woo-Rippe KW, et al. Variability in glycosylated hemoglobin values in diabetic patients living in long-term care facilities. J Am Med Dir Assoc 2007; 8(8):511–4.

[13] Alam T, Weintraub N, Weinreb J. What is the proper use of hemoglobin A1C monitoring in the elderly? J Am Med Dir Assoc 2006;7(Suppl 3):S60–4.

[14] Joseph J, Koka M, Aronow WS. Prevalence of a hemoglobin A1c less than 7.0%, of a blood pressure less than 130/80 Hg, and of a serum low-density lipoprotein cholesterol less than 100 mg/dl in older patients with diabetes mellitus in an academic nursing home. J Am Med Dir Assoc 2008;9(1):51–4.

[15] Koka M, Joseph J, Aronow WS. Prevalence of adequate and of optimal control of serum low-density lipoprotein cholesterol in an academic nursing home. J Am Med Dir Assoc 2007;8(9):605–6.

[16] Zarowitz BJ, Tangalos EG, Hollenack K, et al. The application of evidence based principles of care in older persons (issue 3): management of diabetes mellitus. J Am Med Dir Assoc 2006;7(4):234–40.

[17] Flaherty JH, Perry HM 3rd, Lynchard GS, et al. Polypharmacy and hospitalization among older home care patients. J Gerontol A Biol Sci Med Sci 2000;55(10):M554–9.

[18] Haas LB. Optimizing insulin use in type 2 diabetes: a role of basal and prandial insulin in long-term care facilities. J Am Med Dir Assoc 2007;8(8):502–10.

[19] Mazza AD, Morley JE. Metabolic syndrome and the older male population. Aging Male 2007;10(1):3–8.

[20] Nisen SE, Wolski K. Effect of rosiglitazone on the risk of myocardial infarction and death from cardiovascular causes. N Engl J Med 2007;356(24):2457–71.

[21] Morley JE. Weight loss in the nursing home. J Am Med Dir Assoc 2007;8(4):201–4.

[22] Tariq SH, Karcic E, Thomas DR, et al. The use of a no-concentrated-sweets diet in the management of type 2 diabetes in nursing home. J Am Diet Assoc 2001;101(12):1463–6.

ELSEVIER
SAUNDERS

CLINICS IN
GERIATRIC
MEDICINE

Clin Geriatr Med 24 (2008) 395–405

Diabetes and Aging: Epidemiologic Overview

John E. Morley, MB, BCh[a,b,*]

[a]*Geriatric Research Education and Clinical Center, St. Louis VA Medical Center,*
1 Jefferson Barracks Drive, 11G, St. Louis, MO 63125, USA
[b]*Geriatric Medicine, Saint Louis University School of Medicine,*
1402 S. Grand Boulevard, Room M238, St. Louis, MO 63104-1079, USA

Diabetes mellitus has long been recognized as a cause of accelerated aging [1,2]. As the understanding of the metabolic syndrome has evolved, it has been recognized that the interaction of a panoply of factors in the presence of insulin resistance results in accelerated aging [3–5]. This article explores the increasing prevalence of diabetes mellitus with aging and how insulin resistance leads to accelerated frailty, disability, hospitalization, institutionalization, and death [6,7].

Diabetes prevalence

During the last 50 years there has been a marked increase in the number of persons in the United States who have diabetes. In 1958 fewer than 2 million in the United States were diabetic, whereas today the number approaches 16 million. There has been a similar increase in diabetes throughout the world, with alarming recent increases in diabetes in developing nations as well as in the developed world [8].

Diabetes mellitus is a disease of older persons: more than half of all diabetics in the United States are over 60 years of age. The prevalence of diabetes mellitus peaks in persons between 65 to 74 years of age [9] (Fig. 1). Twenty percent of men and more than 15% of women 65 to 74 years of age have diabetes. There is a decrease in prevalence rates in persons 75 years and older. It is important to recognize that in 25% to 41% of persons who have diabetes the diagnosis has not been made [10]. Diabetes mellitus is more common in Hispanics (especially those from Mexico),

* Geriatric Medicine, Saint Louis University School of Medicine, 1402 S. Grand Boulevard, Room M238, St. Louis, MO 63104-1079.
E-mail address: morley@slu.edu

0749-0690/08/$ - see front matter. Published by Elsevier Inc.
doi:10.1016/j.cger.2008.03.005 *geriatric.theclinics.com*

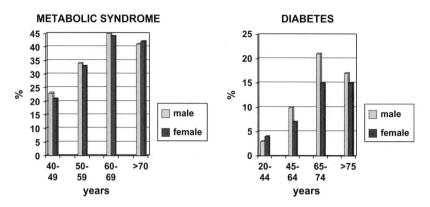

Fig. 1. Prevalence of metabolic syndrome and diabetes by age cohort.

African Americans, and Native Americans. The prevalence of diabetes mellitus in nursing home residents varies, but, in general, about one third of nursing home residents have diabetes [11–13]. In the 2004 National Nursing Home Survey, 24.6% of nursing home residents had diabetes [14]. The prevalence was 35.6% in nonwhites. Nursing home residents who had diabetes took more medicine, had a longer length of stay, and were more likely to have emergency room visits.

In the United States the increased prevalence of diabetes has been linked clearly to the obesity epidemic [15,16]. Although this association is true in middle-aged persons, it is less true in older diabetics, many of whom are not excessively overweight [15]. In an older African American cohort in St. Louis, persons who had diabetes were only mildly more obese than nondiabetics [16]. In a study in Mexico City, 31.9% of diabetics were obese [17].

Prevalence of the metabolic syndrome

The metabolic syndrome was first described by Nicholaes Tulp in Holland in the seventeenth century. He termed it the "hypertriglyceridemia syndrome." In the eighteenth century, G.B. Morgagni described a syndrome that consisted of visceral obesity, hypertension, hyperuricemia, atheroma, and sleep apnea. In the late twentieth century, Gerald Reaven and Ferrannini rediscovered the metabolic syndrome, calling it "syndrome X" and "insulin resistance syndrome," respectively.

The International Diabetes Foundation [18] has defined the metabolic syndrome as

Central obesity: waist circumference
> 94 cm for persons of European origin
> 90 cm for men of Asian origin
>80 cm for women
Plus any two of the following:
• Triglycerides > 1.7 mmol/L (150mg/dL)

- Reduced high-density lipoprotein < 1.03 mmol/L (40 mg/dL) in men or < 1.29 mmol/L (50 mg/dL) in women
- Raised blood pressure > 130 mm Hg systolic and > 85 mm Hg diastolic
- Raised fasting blood glucose > 5.6 nmol/L (100 mg/dL)

As with diabetes mellitus, the prevalence of metabolic syndrome increases with age, peaking at just under 45% in 60- to 69-year-olds [19]. Again, it is slightly more common in men than in women. A study in nursing homes demonstrated that approximately half of the residents had insulin resistance or diabetes, and these conditions were linked to poorer function [20].

The full expression of the metabolic syndrome occurs in persons who have a genetic propensity and who overeat and underexercise. This genetic predisposition and life style lead to visceral obesity with increased tumor necrosis alpha and leptin levels and decreased adiponectin levels [21]. Insulin resistance then leads to hyperinsulinemia. The clinical presentation is hyperglycemia, hypertension, hyperuricemia, alterations in coagulopathy (plasminogen activating inhibitor-1 and fibrinogen), decreased high-density lipoprotein cholesterol, increased triglycerides, increased small, dense low-density lipoprotein cholesterol, nonalcoholic steatohepatitis, and myosteatosis (fat infiltration in muscle). With this constellation of symptoms, it is not surprising that the metabolic syndrome is associated with increased disability [22,23].

Genes and type 2 diabetes

Five recent genome-wide association scans have given insight into the genetic basis of type 2 diabetes [24]. The effect sizes of each allele so far identified are very modest (odds ratio < 1.2). The following potential genes have been identified:

- Insulin-degrading enzyme (*IDE*)
- Homeobox, hematopoietically expressed (*HHEX*): a transcription factor for pancreatic development
- Insulin growth factor 2 mRNA–binding protein (*IGF2BP2*), which plays a role in cell proliferation
- Cyclin-dependent kinase (*CDKN2A/B*), which plays a role in islet proliferation
- Cyclin-dependent kinase 5 regulatory subunit–associated protein 1-like 1 (*CDKAL1*), which reduces insulin secretion
- Scarecrose like 30a8 (*SCL3OA8*) thiazolidinedione (*TZD*) variant, which codes for a pancreatic islet–specific zinc transporter–involved insulin biosynthesis and storage
- Fatso (*FTO*), an obesity locus
- Peroxisome proliferator-activated receptor gamma (*PPAR*-γ), which is involved in insulin resistance
- Potassium channel NJ11 (*KCNJ11*), which codes for a pancreatic beta-cell potassium ATP channel subunit

- Transcription factor 7 like 2 (*TCF7L2*), which is associated with decreased insulin secretion by modulating the WnT signaling pathway

The most interesting finding from these studies is that only two of these genes (*PPAR-γ* and *FTO*) are involved in insulin resistance; the other eight play a role in insulin secretion. This finding confirms, as was pointed out a number of years ago, that type 2 diabetes, particularly in older persons, is more dependent on failure of insulin secretion from the islets of Langerhans than on insulin resistance.

A rare genetic defect associated with diabetes and deafness is the maternally inherited *3243A > G* mutation in mitochondrial DNA [25]. This deficit seems to enhance aging of the pancreatic β cells, leading to a reduced ability of these cells to synthesize insulin.

Diabetes mellitus accelerates aging

At a basic level, diabetes mellitus accelerates the aging process. Diabetes is associated with a decrease in DNA unwinding rate, increased collagen cross-linking, increased capillary basement membrane thickening, increased oxidative damage, and decreased $Na^+K^+ATPase$ activity [26,27].

These basic changes result in increased clinical signs of aging. Cataracts occur 2.5 times more commonly in diabetics than in nondiabetics. Diabetics have accelerated atherosclerosis with increased propensity to have a myocardial infarction, stroke, and peripheral vascular disease [28].

Diabetics have an increased prevalence of cognitive decline [29]. Hyperglycemia has been shown to relate directly to poor memory [30]. Diabetics also are more likely to develop vascular dementia and possibly Alzheimer's disease [31]. Diabetics should be screened regularly for both mild cognitive impairment and dementia using a formal test such as the Saint Louis University Mental Status examination [32].

Diabetics are at increased risk of falling [33] and developing hip fractures [34]. Persons who have diabetes have an increase in functional decline [35] and frailty [36].

Diabetics complain of pain more often than nondiabetics [37], apparently because glucose or advanced glucose end products inhibit the receptors for endorphins.

Like older persons, diabetics are at increased risk for developing incontinence, nocturia, dehydration, and infections. Diabetes mellitus is associated with an increased likelihood of developing pressure ulcers [38].

Alterations of intestinal permeability in persons who have diabetes mellitus increase the propensity for bacterial translocation [39]. This propensity is associated with increased cytokine activation [40]. Increased cytokines have deleterious effects on muscle, red blood cells, the cardiovascular system, the immune system, and cognition [41].

Depression occurs commonly in diabetics and when poorly treated is associated with poor outcomes [15,42]. Overall, diabetes is associated with a decline in quality of life and a decrease in leisure activities, such as reading, gardening, writing letters, and going out socially [43].

Diabetes and testosterone

Testosterone levels decline with aging [44]. Recently, a number of studies have found that testosterone levels are low both in diabetics [45] and in persons who have the metabolic syndrome [46]. An 11-year follow-up study found that low testosterone levels were 1.5 times more prevalent in persons who had metabolic syndrome and were more than twice as prevalent in persons who had diabetes [47].

A number of studies have suggested that testosterone may reduce insulin resistance [48]. In addition testosterone replacement decreases adipose tissue [49]. Smith and colleagues [50] reported that androgen-deprivation therapy for 3 months in men who had prostate cancer resulted in an increase in fat mass and median serum insulin as well as augmentation of central arterial pressure. Recently, androgen-deprivation therapy was shown to be associated with a 1.44-increased risk of diabetes [51]. This increased risk of diabetes produced an increased risk of coronary artery disease, myocardial infarction, and sudden cardiac death. Orchiectomy produced similar effects. Diabetics who have low testosterone or bioavailable testosterone levels may benefit from testosterone replacement [52].

Hypertension and diabetes

The study by the United Kingdom Prospective Diabetes Study Group clearly showed that in middle-aged diabetics treatment of hypertension had the best reduction in myocardial infarction and total mortality [53]. Three major hypertension trials (Systolic Hypertension in the Elderly, Systolic Hypertension in Europe Trial and Heart Outcomes Prevention Evaluation Study) demonstrated that lowering blood pressure in diabetics leads to a reduction in stroke, myocardial infarction, and mortality [54]. In addition, some studies have suggested that treatment with an angiotensin-converting enzyme inhibitor or an angiotensin receptor blocker may decrease the risk of developing diabetes [55]. Control of hypertension often is inadequate in persons who have diabetes [56].

Diabetes and blood pressure

Persons who have diabetes often have autonomic neuropathy, which is a major risk factor for orthostasis [57]. Orthostatic hypotension is associated with falls and increased cardiovascular events and death [58].

Persons who have diabetes mellitus are at increased risk of developing postprandial hypotension [59]. Postprandial hypotension results in increased falls, syncope, myocardial infarction, and death [60]. Although the mechanism by which postprandial hypotension develops is unclear, it is associated with rapid gastric emptying [61]. In addition, the release of vasodilation peptides, such as calcitonin gene-related peptide, seems to play an important role in producing peripheral vasodilatation, which produces the syndrome [62]. Recently, it has been shown that an increase in glucagon-like peptide-I slows gastric emptying and reduces postprandial hypotension [63]. Both the alpha-1-glucosidase inhibitors increase glucagon-like peptide I and can be used to attenuate postprandial hypotension [64,65].

Diabetes and lipids

It is well recognized that hyperlipidemia interacts synergistically with diabetes to produce cardiovascular disease [66]. A recent meta-analysis has shown that the use of statins has beneficial effects in the treatment of persons between 70 and 80 years of age [67]. There are few data in persons over the age of 80 years, although the Prospective Study of Provastatin in Elderly at Risk study failed to find an effect of pravastatin on mortality, function, or mental status in persons over the age of 80 years [68]. The major negative effects of cholesterol seem to be associated with the occurrence of small, dense low-density lipoprotein, and awareness of that association may help in the decision of whether to use statins in the old-old.

Recent studies have shown that increasing fish and fish oils in the diet has a positive effect on hyperlipidemia [69]. Lipid control in persons who have diabetes living in nursing homes often is inadequate [70,71].

Diabetes and weight loss

With aging many older persons develop anorexia [72], which has been characterized as "the anorexia of aging" [73]. Weight loss has been associated consistently with poor outcomes in older persons. A single study in older diabetics found that weight loss was related to an increased hazard of death [74]. Studies in nursing home residents have failed to demonstrate a benefit of diabetic diets [75].

These findings need to be contrasted with three studies in middle-aged and young-old persons that showed that lifestyle interventions consisting of diet and exercise consistently slowed the onset of diabetes mellitus [76,77]. This finding also was true in persons aged over 60 years, and metformin failed to be protective in this group [78]. The author and his colleagues strongly believe that diet modification needs to be associated with exercise (aerobic, resistance, and balance exercises) if it is to have positive outcomes [79].

Reasons for maintenance of euglycemia in older diabetics

There are a variety of reasons to maintain euglycemia in older persons:

- Prevention of hyperglycemic comas
- Prevention of long-term complications
- Prevention of glucose toxicity
    Accelerated aging
    Trace mineral deficiency
    Infection
    Dehydration
    Incontinence/nocturia
    Reduction in pain perception
    Cognitive dysfunction

Although the most common hyperglycemic coma with type 2 diabetes is hyperosmolar coma, older persons often have a mixed hyperosmolar/ketotic coma [80]. Lactic acid coma also is more common in older persons. These comas often are precipitated by an inciting event, such as a myocardial infarction. In addition, there is increasing evidence that control of excessive glycemia improves outcomes in older persons who are hospitalized, especially for surgical procedures [81].

Age conspires with poorly controlled diabetes mellitus to accelerate the long-term complications of retinopathy, nephropathy, and neuropathy. In older persons, treatment of diabetes decreases the rate of progression of retinopathy [82].

Hyperglycemia accelerates the aging process by producing increased advanced glucose end products, oxidative damage, and DNA breaks [27]. The physiologic age of the average diabetic is 10 years older than the person's chronologic age.

Hyperglycemia is an ideal environment for bacterial growth. Diabetics are more likely than nondiabetics to have recurrence of tuberculosis [83]. Diabetics often have atypical infections such as mucomycosis and candidiasis [84].

Hyperglycemia causes an increase in urinary fluid loss leading to an increase in incontinence and nocturia [85]. In addition, the hyperosmolar diuresis leads to dehydration. This diuresis also leads to loss of trace elements, causing hypomagnesemia and zinc deficiency [86]. Zinc deficiency can lead to worsening hyperglycemia immune dysfunction and pressure ulcers [87].

Persons who have diabetes mellitus complain of more pain than other persons. Hyperglycemia leads to an increased perception of pain [37] that seems to be caused by glucose interfering with the endorphin receptors.

Numerous studies in humans and animals have demonstrated that diabetes is associated with cognitive dysfunction [88]. Lowering glucose levels improves cognitive function [30]. Dementia is more common in persons who have diabetes mellitus [89].

Overall, all these issues argue for the importance of adequate control of hyperglycemia in older persons who have diabetes mellitus.

References

[1] Mazza AD, Morley JE. Update on diabetes in the elderly and the application of current therapeutics. J Am Med Dir Assoc 2007;8:489–92.

[2] Morley JE. An overview of diabetes mellitus in older persons. Clin Geriatr Med 1999;15: 211–24.

[3] Mazza AD, Morley JE. Metabolic syndrome and the older male population. Aging Male 2007;10:3–8.

[4] Morley JE. Diabetes mellitus: a major disease of older persons. J Gerontol A Biol Sci Med Sci 2000;55:M255–6.

[5] Blaum CS, West NA, Haan MN. Is the metabolic syndrome, with or without diabetes, associated with progressive disability in older Mexican Americans? J Gerontol A Biol Sci Med Sci 2007;62:766–73.

[6] Morley JE, Kim MJ, Haren MT, et al. Frailty and the aging male. Aging Male 2005;8: 135–40.

[7] Abellan van Kan G, Rolland YM, Morley JE, et al. Frailty: toward a clinical definition. J Am Med Dir Assoc 2008;9:71–2.

[8] Kim MJ, Rolland Y, Cepeda O, et al. Diabetes mellitus in older men. Aging Male 2006;9: 139–47.

[9] Resnick HE, Harris MI, Brock DB, et al. American Diabetes Association diabetes diagnostic criteria, advancing age, and cardiovascular disease risk profiles: results from the Third National Health and Nutrition Examination Survey. Diabetes Care 2000;23:176–80.

[10] Morley JE, Perry HM 3rd. The management of diabetes mellitus in older individuals. Drugs 1991;41:548–65.

[11] Mooradian AD, Osterweil D, Petrasek D, et al. Diabetes mellitus in elderly nursing home patients. A survey of clinical characteristics and management. J Am Geriatr Soc 1988;36: 391–6.

[12] Joseph J, Koka M, Aronow WS. Prevalence of a hemoglobin A1c less than 7.0%, of a blood pressure less than 130/80 Hg, and of a serum low-density lipoprotein cholesterol less than 100 mg/dl in older patients with diabetes mellitus in an academic nursing home. J Am Med Dir Assoc 2008;9:51–4.

[13] Haas LB. Optimizing insulin use in type 2 diabetes: role of basal and prandial insulin in long-term care facilities. J Am Med Dir Assoc 2007;8:511–4.

[14] Resnick HE, Heineman J, Stone R, et al. Diabetes in nursing homes: United States 2004. Diabetes Care 2007;31:287–8.

[15] Rosenthal MJ, Fajardo M, Gilmore S, et al. Hospitalization and mortality of diabetes in older adults. A 3-year prospective study. Diabetes Care 1998;21:231–5.

[16] Miller DK, Lui LY, Petty HM 3rd, et al. Reported and measured physical functioning in older inner-city diabetic African-Americans. J Gerontol A BIol Sci Med Sci 1999;54: M230–6.

[17] Rodriguez-Saldana J, Morley JE, Reynoso MT, et al. Diabetes mellitus in a subgroup of older Mexicans: prevalence, association with cardiovascular risk factors, functional and cognitive impairment, and mortality. J Am Geriatr Soc 2002;50:111–6.

[18] Sandhofer A, Iglseder B, Paulweber B, et al. Comparison of different definitions of the metabolic syndrome. Eur J Clin Invest 2007;37:109–16.

[19] Ford ES, Giles WH, Dietz WH. Prevalence of the metabolic syndrome among US adults: findings from the third National Health and Nutrition Examination Survey. JAMA 2002; 287:356–9.

ELSEVIER
SAUNDERS

CLINICS IN
GERIATRIC
MEDICINE

Clin Geriatr Med 24 (2008) 407–435

Diabetic Neuropathy in Older Adults

Aaron I. Vinik, MD, PhD[a],[*],
Elsa S. Strotmeyer, PhD, MPH[b],
Abhijeet A. Nakave, MBBS[a],
Chhaya V. Patel, MBBS[a]

[a]*Strelitz Diabetes Institutes, Department of Internal Medicine, Eastern Virginia
Medical School, 855 West Brambleton Avenue, Norfolk, VA 23510, USA*
[b]*Center for Aging and Population Health, Department of Epidemiology,
Graduate School of Public Health, University of Pittsburgh, 130 North Bellefield Avenue,
Pittsburgh, PA 15213, USA*

Diabetic neuropathies (DN) encompass a wide range of nerve abnormalities and are common, with prevalence rates reported between 5% and 100%, depending on the diagnostic criteria [1–3]. DN affect both peripheral and autonomic nervous systems and cause considerable morbidity and mortality in both Type I and Type II diabetic patients. DN are the most common forms of neuropathy; they account for more hospitalizations than all other diabetic complications combined, and are responsible for 50% to 75% of nontraumatic amputations [4,5]. In older adults who have diabetes, peripheral neuropathies are especially troublesome because of their detrimental effects on stability, sensorimotor function, gait, and activities of daily living (ADL) [6–8]. In the United States for 1999 to 2000, 28% of adults aged 70 to 79 years and 35% of adults aged more than 80 years had peripheral neuropathy, based on a simple screen for reduced sensation at the foot [9]. In this article, the authors present and discuss the most recent approaches to the treatment of the common forms of diabetic neuropathy, including symmetric, focal, and diffuse neuropathies (Box 1) (Fig. 1). We also provide the reader with algorithms for recognition and management of common pain and entrapment syndromes, and a global approach to recognition of syndromes requiring specialized treatments based upon our improved understanding of their etiopathogenesis. A comprehensive

Portions of the text are from Witzke KA, Vinik AI. Diabetic neuropathy in older adults. Rev Endocr Metab Disord 2005;6(2):117–27; with permission.
* Corresponding author.
E-mail address: vinikai@evms.edu (A.I. Vinik).

doi:10.1016/j.cger.2008.03.011
geriatric.theclinics.com

Box 1. Classification of diabetic neuropathy

Focal neuropathies
- Mononeuritis
- Entrapment syndromes

Diffuse neuropathies
- Proximal motor (amyotrophy)
    Coexisting chronic inflammatory demyelinating
        polyneuropathy (CIDP)
    Monoclonal gammopathy of undetermined significance
        (MGUS)
    Circulating GM1 antibodies and antibodies to neuronal
        cells
    Inflammatory vasculitis

Generalized symmetric polyneuropathies
- Acute sensory
- Autonomic
- Chronic sensorimotor distal polyneuropathy (DPN)
    Large fiber
    Small fiber

Note Clinicians should be alert for treatable neuropathies occurring in diabetic patients, including CIDP, monoclonal gammopathy, vitamin B_{12} deficiency etc.

Data from Thomas PK. Classification, differential diagnosis, and staging of diabetic peripheral neuropathy. Diabetes 1997;46(Suppl 2):S54–7 and Vinik A. Diagnosis and management of diabetic neuropathy. Clin Geriatr Med 1999;15:294.

---

evaluation of autonomic neuropathy is beyond the scope of this article, but the reader is referred to two excellent reviews on this topic [10,11].

Pathogenic mechanisms

Figs. 2 and 3 show our current view on the pathogenesis of diabetes. Fig. 2 depicts multiple etiologies, as discussed above, including metabolic, vascular, autoimmune, oxidative, and nitrosative stress, and neurohormonal growth-factor deficiency. Inflammation is more clearly involved in the specific inflammatory neuropathies such as vasculitic and granulomatous disease than in diabetic neuropathy per se [12], though this has not been studied in age-related neuropathies. P- and E-selectin, activated during the inflammatory process, predict the decline in peripheral nerve function among diabetic patients [13]. Impaired blood flow and endoneurial microvasculopathy, mainly thickening of the blood vessel wall or occlusion, play critical roles in the pathogenesis of diabetic neuropathy. Metabolic disturbances in the presence of an underlying genetic predisposition cause reduced nerve perfusion. Animal and human studies alike have shown major

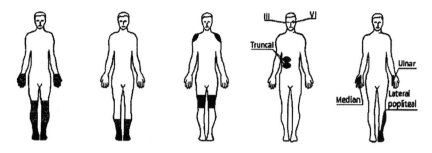

Large fiber Neuropathy	Small fiber Neuropathy	Proximal motor Neuropathy	Acute mono Neuropathies	Pressure Palsies
Sensory loss: 0→ +++ (Touch, vibration) Pain: + → +++ Tendon reflex: N → ↓↓↓ Motor deficit 0 → +++	Sensory loss: 0 → + (thermal , allodynia) Pain: + → +++ . Tendon reflex: N → ↓ Motor deficit: 0	Sensory loss: 0 → + Pain: + → +++ Tendon reflex: ↓↓ Proximal Motor deficit: + → +++.	Sensory loss: 0 → + Pain: + → +++ Tendon reflex: N Motor deficit: + → +++	Sensory loss in Nerve distribution: + → +++ Pain: + → ++ Tendon reflex: N Motor deficit: + → +++

Fig. 1. Different clinical presentations of diabetic neuropathy. (*From* Vinik AI, Park TS, Stansberry KB, et al. Diabetologia 2000;43:960; with permission.)

defects arising from chronic hyperglycemia and altered lipid metabolism [14]. Oxidative stress-related mechanisms are also important in vascular dysfunction, and tend to increase vasoconstriction. These alterations in blood flow patterns appear to be important in the understanding of the arterio-venous shunting seen in vasa nervorum, which may occur in part because of autonomic nerve dysfunction. Sensory and local autonomic nerve function deficits appear to predominate in patients who have critical limb ischemia

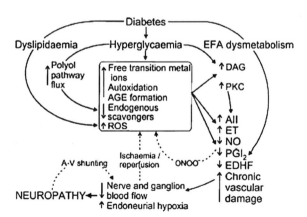

Fig. 2. Pathogenesis of diabetic neuropathy based upon oxidative/nitrosative stress and metabolic processes. AII, angiotensin II; A-V, arteriovenous; EFA, essential fatty acid; ET, endothelin-1; ONOO⁻, peroxynitrite; PGI₂, prostacyclin; PKC, protein kinase C. (*From* Cameron NE, Eaton SEM, Cotter MA, et al. Vascular factors and metabolic interactions in the pathogenesis of diabetic neuropathy. Diabetologia 2001;44:1973–88; with permission.)

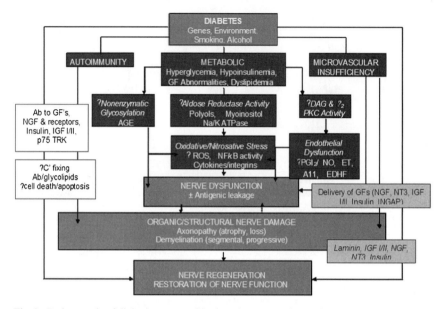

Fig. 3. Pathogenesis of diabetic neuropathies based upon autoimmunity, metabolic and microvascular insufficiency. Ab, antibody; AGE, advance glycation end products; C¢, complement; DAG, diacylglycerol; ET, endothelin; EDHF, endothelium-derived hyperpolarizing factor; GF, growth factor; IGF, insulinlike growth factor; NFkB, nuclear factor kB; NGF, nerve growth factor; NO, nitric oxide; NT3, neurotropin 3; PKC, protein kinase C; PGI2, prostaglandin I2; ROS, reactive oxygen species; TRK, tyrosine kinase. (*From* Vinik A, Casellini DC, Nakave A, et al. Chapter 35. Diabetic neuropathies. 2007; with permission. Available at: http://endotext.org/diabetes/diabetes35/diabetesframe35.htm. Accessed March 10, 2008.)

[15]. Improving blood flow to tissues may improve nerve conduction velocity in diabetic neuropathy [16]. Oxidative and nitrosative stress and inflammation are implicated in several neurodegenerative disorders, including Alzheimer's disease and amyotrophic lateral sclerosis (ALS) [17]. Oxidative stress is indicated as a contributor in diabetic neuropathy [18]. It is greater in diabetic patients before development of peripheral neuropathy, and particularly in those who have peripheral neuropathy [19]. Potentially, similar mechanisms play a role in the peripheral nerve with aging, because aging [20] and Type II diabetes [21–25] are associated with an increased levels of subclinical systemic inflammatory markers, such as cytokines interleukin (IL)-6 and tumor necrosis factor (TN)F-α, and acute phase proteins such as C-reactive protein (CRP).

Clinical presentation and diagnosis

Focal neuropathies (mononeuropathies and entrapment syndromes)

Mononeuropathies occur primarily in older adults. Their onset is generally acute and associated with pain, and they heal spontaneously, usually within 6 to 8 weeks. These neuropathies are caused by vascular obstruction, typically in the cranial nerves III, VI, and VII, ulnar, median, and peroneal. Mononeuropathies must be distinguished from entrapment syndromes, which start slowly, progress, and persist without intervention (Table 1).

Common entrapment sites in diabetic patients involve the median, ulnar, and peroneal nerves, the lateral cutaneous nerve of the thigh, and the tibial nerve in the tarsal canal. Their onset is gradual and is usually limited to a single nerve [26]. Carpal tunnel syndrome is the most common entrapment syndrome, affecting one in three diabetic patients [27]. It occurs three times more frequently in patients who have diabetes compared with the normal healthy population [28], and may be related to diabetic cheiroarthropathy, repeated undetected trauma, metabolic changes, or an accumulation of fluid or edema within the confined space of the carpal tunnel [29]. Surgical treatment of entrapment syndrome neuropathies is effective, but the decision to proceed with surgery should be based on severity of symptoms, appearance of motor weakness, and failure of nonsurgical treatment.

Diffuse neuropathies (proximal motor neuropathies)

Proximal motor neuropathy can be clinically identified based on proximal muscle weakness and muscle wasting. It may be symmetric or asymmetric in distribution, and is sometimes associated with pain in the lateral aspect of the thigh. Patients usually present with weakness of the iliopsoas, obturator, and adductor muscles, together with relative preservation of the

Table 1

Comparison of features of mononeuropathies, entrapment syndromes and distal symmetric polyneuropathy

Feature	Mononeuropathy	Entrapment syndrome	Neuropathy
Onset	Sudden	Gradual	Gradual
Pattern	Single nerve, but may be multiple	Single nerve exposed to trauma	Distal symmetric poly neuropathy
Nerves involved	Cranial nerves (CN) III, VI, VII, ulnar, median, peroneal	Median, ulnar, peroneal, medial and lateral plantar	Mixed, motor, sensory, autonomic
Natural history	Resolves spontaneously	Progressive	Progressive
Treatment	Symptomatic	Rest, splints, local steroids, diuretics, surgery	Tight glycemic control, pregabalin, duloxetine, antioxidants, "nutrinerve," research drugs
Distribution of sensory loss	Area supplied by the nerve	Area supplied beyond the site of entrapment	Distal and symmetric. "Glove and stocking" distribution

From Vinik A, Casellini DC, Nakave A, et al. Chapter 35. Diabetic neuropathies. 2007; with permission. Available at: http://endotext.org/diabetes/diabetes35/diabetesframe35.htm. Accessed March 10, 2008.

gluteus maximus and minimus, and hamstrings [30,31]. Those affected have great difficulty rising out of chair unaided, although heel or toe standing is surprisingly good. In the classic form of diabetic proximal motor neuropathy, axonal loss is the predominant process, and the condition coexists with distal symmetric polyneuropathy [32]. Electrophysiologic evaluation reveals lumbosacral plexopathy [33]. Common features include

- Primarily affects the elderly
- Onset may be gradual or acute
- Begins with pain in the thighs and hips or buttocks
- Pain followed by significant weakness of the proximal muscles of the lower limbs with inability to rise from the sitting position (positive Gower's maneuver)
- Begins unilaterally and spreads bilaterally
- Coexists with DPN
- Spontaneous muscle fasciculation, or provoked by percussion

Proximal motor neuropathy is now recognized as being secondary to a variety of causes unrelated to diabetes, but which occur more frequently in patients who have diabetes than in the general population. It includes patients who have CIDP, MGUS, circulating GM1 antibodies and antibodies to neuronal cells, and inflammatory vasculitis [34,35]. Vinik [36] (Fig. 4) found that almost half of patients who have proximal neuropathies have a vasculitis, and all but 9% have CIDP, MGUS, or a ganglioside antibody syndrome [36,37]. Sharma and colleagues [38] examined over 1000 patients who had neurologic disorders and found that CIDP was 11 times more frequent among diabetic than nondiabetic patients (Fig. 5).

In contrast, if demyelination predominates and the motor deficit affects proximal and distal muscle groups, the diagnosis of CIDP should be considered. It is important to divide proximal syndromes into these two subcategories because the CIDP variant responds dramatically to intervention [36,38,39], with IVIG, plasmaphereis, steroids and immunosuppresive

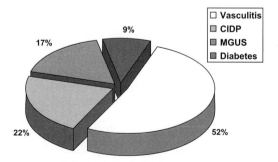

Fig. 4. Percentage of different disabling peripheral neuropathy in older adults. MGUS, monoclonal gammopathy of uncertain significance. (*From* Sharma K, Cross J, Farronay O, et al. Demyelinating neuropathy in diabetes mellitus. Arch Neurol 2002;59:758–65; with permission.)

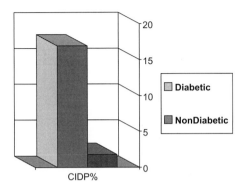

Fig. 5. Frequency of CIDP. There is an 11 fold greater frequency of CIDP in patients with diabetes. (*From* Sharma K, Cross J, Farronay O, et al. Demyelinating neuropathy in diabetes mellitus. Arch Neurol 2002;59:758–65; with permission.)

agents [36] whereas proximal motor neuropathy runs its own course over months to years. Until more evidence is available, we consider them as separate syndromes.

These conditions should be distinguished from spinal stenosis syndromes common in older individuals, which occur because of: (1) encroachment on nerve roots as they emerge from the spinal cord, (2) osteophytes that narrow joint space and cause compression, (3) hypertrophy of the ligamentum flavum caused by aging, (4) disk dehydration caused by aging, and (5) arachnoiditis. If compression occurs at the level of T12 and L1/2, the vascular system may be involved. This often causes claudication during downhill walking, and is relieved with spinal flexion. Nerve root compression is more typical at L5/S1, and thus in difficult cases it may be necessary to obtain an MRI of the lumbosacral spine. Diagnosis is critical because therapy may range from simple physical therapy to surgical decompression if symptoms are severe or if motor paralysis exists.

Chronic sensorimotor distal polyneuropathy

Chronic sensorimotor DPN is the most common and widely recognized form of diabetic neuropathy. The onset is usually insidious, following stress or initiation of therapy for diabetes. DPN may be either sensory or motor, and may involve small fibers, large fibers, or both [43]. Initial neurologic evaluation should focus on detection of the specific part of the nervous system affected by diabetes. Most patients who have DPN have a combination of both large and small nerve fiber involvement (Fig. 6).

Large fiber neuropathies

A majority of neuropathies in older adults involve large fibers. Large fiber neuropathies may involve sensory or motor nerves, and most patients will present with a "glove and stocking" distribution of sensory loss [44].

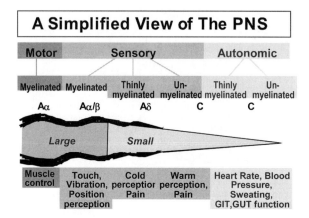

Fig. 6. Schematic presentation of the physiologic function of different nerve fibers: Aα fibers are large myelinated fibers, in charge of motor functions and muscle control. Aα/β fibers are also large myelinated fibers, with sensory functions such as perception to touch, vibration, and position. Aδ fibers are small myelinated fibers, in charge of pain stimuli and cold perception. C fibers can be myelinated or unmyelinated and have both sensory (warm perception and pain) and autonomic functions (blood pressure and heart rate regulation, sweating, etc). GIT, gastrointestinal tract; GUT, genitourinary tract. (*From* Vinik A, Casellini DC, Nakave A, et al. Chapter 35. Diabetic neuropathies. 2007; with permission. Available at: http://endotext.org/diabetes/diabetes35/diabetesframe35.htm. Accessed March 10, 2008.)

These tend to be the neuropathies of signs rather than symptoms. They are manifested by reduced vibration (often the first objective evidence of neuropathy) and position sense, weakness, muscle wasting, and depressed tendon reflexes. Early in the course of the neuropathic process, multifocal sensory loss might also be found (Table 2). The symptoms may be minimal, such as a sensation of walking on cotton, floors feeling "strange," inability to turn the pages of a book, or inability to discriminate among coins. In some patients, severe distal muscle weakness can accompany the sensory loss, resulting in an inability to stand on the toes or heels.

Little is known, however, at the clinical and population levels about the role of age-related loss in peripheral nerve function in sarcopenia and loss of

Table 2
Decline in neurologic function between 20–80 years

Function	Percent dysfunction
Vibratory sensation	97%
Stability (Rombergism)	32%
Handwriting speed	30%
Handgrip strength	22%
Ankle jerk	9%
Ataxia (finger nose test)	8%
Pain perception	0%

Data from Refs. [40–42].

strength associated with aging. Loss of lean mass, or sarcopenia, is thought to account for much of the loss of strength and function in older adults [45,46]. In addition to lower mass, aging muscle is characterized by loss of muscle fibers, predominantly type 2 fast-twitch fibers, and an increase in grouping or "clustering" of type 1 fibers [47]. These changes are thought to be caused in part by disuse atrophy and in part to dropout of the anterior horn motor neuron at the level of the spinal cord. When the motor neuron is lost with disease (polio, ALS) or aging, remaining motor neurons can sprout new dendritic connections to "orphaned" muscle fibers. This reinnervation process may be responsible for the increase in grouping of type 1 fibers, and may limit regaining type 2 fibers after loss caused by atrophy. Although the innervation of muscle tissue is essential to its function, very little is known about the relative contribution of peripheral nerve function to muscle function and functional decline in community-dwelling older adults. In diabetes, severe peripheral neuropathy is quite clearly related to muscle atrophy [48]. By MRI scanning, diabetic neuropathy in Type I diabetes is associated with a 50% reduction in muscle volume, with a high correlation between neuropathy score and muscle volume ($r = -0.75$, $P < .001$) [49]. Given the known atrophy and denervation in the pathophysiologic description of muscle aging, it is remarkable how little is known at the clinical and population levels about the role of age-related loss in nerve function in the age-related loss of muscle mass and strength. This neurogenic process may be a critical link in the pathogenesis of sarcopenia and mobility loss in old age.

Older adults who have large fiber neuropathies have difficulty stabilizing their bodies when walking on irregular surfaces, with concomitant impairment in reaction time and balance [6]. This lack of peripheral sensory input increases the risk of falling and fracture in these patients. In the Women's Health and Aging study, women who had diabetes reported difficulty in performing 14 of 15 daily tasks, which included walking two to three blocks, lifting 10 pounds, using a telephone, and bathing [7]. Failure to perform basic activities of daily living readily compromises an individual's independence and quality of life (QOL), which increases mortality and morbidity in this susceptible population [50]. The Norfolk QOL tool is used to measure patients' perception of the effects of diabetes and diabetic neuropathy [50].

Epidemiologic studies have found that older adults who have poor peripheral nerve function have worse physical performance, balance, muscle density, and bone density [22,23,51–53]. Most of these associations were independent of diabetes status. A twofold higher prospective decline in motor performance exists for older adults who have distal symmetric neuropathy [54]. Clinical consequences of higher fall and fracture rates are also evident in older adults who have peripheral nerve impairments. In a prospective cohort aged 70 years and older, those who had loss of touch sensation in their feet had a 2.5 times greater risk of major injurious falls, including fractures, joint dislocations, lacerations requiring sutures, and intracranial injuries

[55]. In the Study of Osteoporotic Fractures, recurrent falling was related to worse vibration sense (age-adjusted OR = 1.12, 95% CI, 1.05–1.19) and loss of touch sensation (age-adjusted OR = 1.58, 95% CI, 1.34–1.87) in older women [56].

In recent years, several inexpensive devices have been developed for the assessment of somatosensory function, including vibration, thermal energy, and light-touch perception. These instruments allow for the noninvasive assessment of cutaneous sensory functions, which correlate with specific neural fiber function. In addition to the above modalities, quantitative sensory tests (QST) are available for the assessment of pain threshold and cutaneous current perception [43]. Clinical manifestations of large fiber neuropathies include

- Impaired vibration perception and position sense
- Depressed tendon reflexes
- Dull (like a toothache), crushing, or cramplike pain in the bones of the feet
- Sensory ataxia (waddling like a duck)
- Wasting of small muscles of the feet with hammertoes and weakness of hands and feet
- Shortening of the Achilles tendon with equinus.
- Increased blood flow to the foot (hot foot) with increased risk of Charcot neuroarthropathy.

Small fiber neuropathies

Small nerve fiber dysfunction usually occurs early and is often present without objective signs or electrophysiologic evidence of nerve damage [43]. It manifests first in the lower limbs with symptoms of pain and hyperalgesia, followed by a loss of thermal sensitivity and reduced light-touch and pinprick sensation [57]. Small unmyelinated C-fibers control pain sensation, warm thermal perception, and autonomic function. A patient who has early damage to these nerves may experience burning, dysesthetic pain, often accompanied by hyperalgesia, and allodynia. This pain is distinct from that of large fiber neuropathy, in which the pain is usually described as deep and "gnawing." Because peripheral sympathetic nerve fibers are also composed of small, unmyelinated C-fibers, it is not surprising that pain is improved with sympathetic blocking agents (eg, beta-blockers, calcium channel blockers).

It should be noted that dry, cracked skin and impaired skin blood flow in the feet, together with impaired sympathetic regulation of sweat glands and arteriovenous (AV) shunt vessels in the feet, create a favorable environment for bacteria. In the absence of pain, which occurs with the depletion of substance P, patients may be led to believe that their neuropathy has subsided, when in fact it is progressing. These patients may also display decreased thermal pain thresholds, which may be caused in part to the decrease in nerve growth factor (NGF) that maintains small fiber neurons. The clinical manifestations of small fiber neuropathies are summarized below:

- Prominent pain: burning and superficial and associated with allodynia; ie, interpretation of all stimuli as painful (eg, touch)
- Hypoalgesia late in the condition
- Defective autonomic function with decreased sweating, dry skin, impaired vasomotion and blood flow, and cold feet
- Intact reflexes, motor strength
- Silent electrophysiology
- Reduced sensitivity to 1.0 g Semmes Weinstein monofilament and pricking sensation using the Waardenberg wheel or similar instrument
- Abnormal thresholds for warm thermal perception, neurovascular function, pain, quantitative sudorimetry, and quantitative autonomic function tests
- Increased risk of foot ulceration and subsequent gangrene

Differential diagnosis

Diabetes as the cause of neuropathy is diagnosed by exclusion of various other causes of neuropathy. In those patients who have diabetes and neuropathy who present with symptoms of distal symmetric sensorimotor deficit, differential diagnosis should include: hereditary sensory neuropathies, B_{12} and folate deficiency, syphilis, Lyme disease, neuropathy associated with IgM monoclonal gammopathy of undetermined significance (IgM MGUS neuropathy), other paraneoplastic conditions, autoimmune diseases, and toxic neuropathies. In patients who have one or more motor neurologic syndromes, chronic motor neuropathies, acute inflammatory demyelinating polyneuropathy (AIDP), CIDP, and immunoglobulin (Ig)G and IgA MGUS neuropathies should actively be sought (Table 3).

Recent evidence supports an autoimmune etiology for neuropathy in AIDS, Lyme disease, AIDP, CIDP, multifocal motor neuropathy, MGUS neuropathies, and even diabetic polyneuropathy [29,44]. Hence, an intensive workup for humoral immune mechanisms should be performed. If any of these conditions are found, the appropriate therapeutic regime for the specific disease must be instituted before embarking on a regime of diabetic neuropathy management. It is not always possible to determine the exact cause of neuropathy if monoclonal gammopathy and diabetes coexist in the same patient. A course of intravenous immunoglobulin (IVIg) or immunosuppression should be attempted, depending on the class of monoclonal antibody.

Nerve tissue biopsy may be helpful for excluding other causes of neuropathy and in the determination of predominant pathologic changes in patients who have complex clinical findings as a means of dictating choice of treatment [39,58]. The authors' laboratory performs nerve biopsies only when

Table 3
Differential diagnosis of distal symmetric polyneuropathy

Type	Syndrome
Congenital/familial	Charcot-Marie-Tooth
Traumatic	Entrapment syndromes
Inflammatory	Sarcoidosis
	Leprosy
	Lyme disease
	HIV
Neoplastic	Carcinoma–paraneoplastic syndromes
	Myeloma, amyloid
	Reticuloses, leukemias, lymphomas
Metabolic/endocrine	Diabetes mellitus
	Uremia
	Pernicious anemia (B12 deficiency)
	Hypothyroidism
	Porphyria (acute intermittent)
Vascular	Diabetes, vasculitis
Toxic	Alcohol
	Heavy metals (lead, mercury, arsenic)
	Hydrocarbons, chemotherapeutic drugs
Autoimmune	Diabetes
	Phospholipid antibody syndrome
	Chronic inflammatory demyelinating neuropathy
	Multifocal motor neuropathy
	Guillain-Barre syndrome

noninvasive neurologic procedures fail to provide an answer or when extensive evaluation is necessary for scientific purposes [58]. We expect a further increase in our dependence on histopathologic and ultrastructural examination of nerve tissue for differentiation of neuropathic syndromes, as our knowledge of pathophysiologic and clinical complexity among diabetic neuropathic variants increases. Fig. 7 depicts a diagnostic algorithm for the assessment of neurologic deficit and classification of neuropathic syndromes.

Charcot neuroarthropathy

Charcot neuroarthropathy is a progressive condition associated with prolonged neuropathy and characterized by pathologic fracture, joint dislocation, and if left untreated, disabling joint deformity. The most common location for Charcot is in the foot. The prevailing theory of Charcot progression suggests that autonomic neuropathy causes increased blood flow to the extremities, which increases bone resorption and causes osteopenia. Subsequent motor neuropathies cause muscular imbalance, which places abnormal stress on the affected extremity. Sensory neuropathies prevent the patient from sensing abnormal changes in the joints and bones, which may occur because of minor trauma, such as during walking [59]. It is further hypothesized that Achilles tendon shortening caused by destruction of

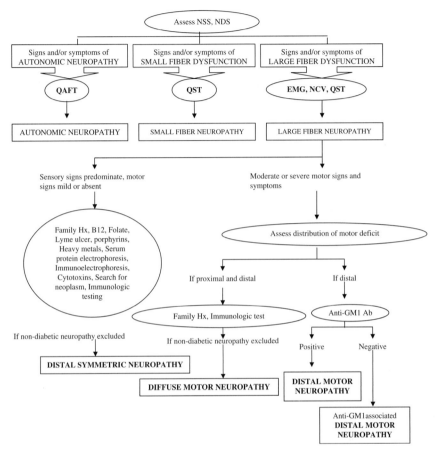

Fig. 7. A diagnostic algorithm for assessment of neurologic deficit and classification of neuropathic syndrome. NSS; neurologic symptom score, NDS; nerve disability score, QST; quantitative sensory test, QAFT; quantitative autonomic function test; EMG, electromyography; NCV, nerve conduction velocity; Hx, history; Ab, antibody. (*From* Vinik AI, Mitchell BD, Leichter SB, et al. Epidemiology of the complications of diabetes. In: Leslie RDG, Robbins DC, editors. Diabetes: clinical science in practice. Cambridge [United Kingdom]: Cambridge University Press; 1995. p. 221–87; reprinted with the permission of Cambridge University Press.)

collagen fibers may be caused by accumulation of advanced glycation end products (AGEs) [60,61].

Patients who have Charcot neuroarthropathy may present acutely with severe pain (or no pain if severe sensory neuropathy), a warm-to-hot swollen foot with increased skin blood flow (despite decreased warm sensory perception and vibration detection), and possible radiographic evidence of osteopenia. The acute Charcot foot can mimic cellulitis or, less commonly, deep vein thrombosis, so these should be first investigated. It should also be noted that radiographic findings can be normal in the acute phase, with subsequent films showing severe subluxation or fracture. Strict immobilization and protection of the foot using a total contact cast is the recommended approach to treating acute Charcot. Pain and inflammation respond to bisphosphonates (eg, slow IV pamidronate infusion over 12 hours) within 3 to 4 weeks [62]. It is worth noting that oral bisphosphonates may cause esophageal dysfunction and increase the risk of obstruction and perforation. Achilles tendon shortening producing equinus is correctable by surgical lengthening, and may prevent further progression. Patient education, protective footwear, and routine foot care are required to prevent further complications such as foot ulceration. In cases of severe joint and bony destruction, reconstructive surgery is effective in salvaging the limb and improving mobility and QOL [50].

Management of neuropathy

The high prevalence of certain subclinical diseases in the elderly may be associated with declines in peripheral nerve function. Importantly, these conditions are modifiable, so early intervention on these risk factors may prevent peripheral nerve function declines and the subsequent clinical consequences associated with peripheral neuropathy. Vitamin B12 deficiency is a known cause of clinical neuropathy [63]; however, the impact of marginally poor vitamin B12 levels, found in between 22% and 35% of community-dwelling older adults [64–66], on peripheral nerve decline is unknown. This has clear clinical implications for defining B12 replacement criteria [67]. Nearly all peripheral arterial disease (PAD) in the elderly is subclinical, with 98% asymptomatic [68]. An Italian study in community-dwelling elderly found an association of subclinical PAD and poor nerve function [69]. This finding is of particular importance because 12% of older adults aged 70 to 79 years and 22% of those aged 80 years or more in the United States have subclinical PAD. Subclinical PAD is underappreciated clinically, but is highly preventable [70,71].

The metabolic syndrome represents another prevalent risk factor for peripheral nerve impairments in the elderly. Prevalence of the metabolic syndrome in the United States is greater than 40% in adults aged 60 years or older [72]. It is a risk factor for peripheral neuropathy among diabetic adults [73,74]. In the Cardiovascular Health Study of older adults, participants who had normal glucose metabolism or a mildly elevated impaired fasting glucose (IFG) had lower heart rate variability (HRV), a marker of cardiovascular autonomic neuropathy, in the presence of two or more components of the metabolic syndrome [72]. In addition to the reduction of blood glucose levels, prevention and treatment of the other components of the metabolic syndrome (obesity, lipid abnormalities, and high blood pressure) could be targeted to prevent peripheral nerve declines in older adults.

Once the diagnosis of neuropathy has been made, therapy to reduce symptoms and prevent further progression should be initiated. Diabetic patients who have large fiber neuropathies are incoordinate and ataxic and are 17 times more likely to fall than their non-neuropathic counterparts

[75]. Older subjects have a higher incidence of neuropathy than younger subjects, especially involving large fibers. It is vitally important to improve strength and balance in the patient who has large fiber neuropathy. Older adults who have or do not have neuropathy can benefit from high intensity strength training by increasing muscle strength, improving coordination and balance, and thus reducing fall and fracture risk [76,77]. Low impact activities that emphasize muscular strength and coordination and challenge the vestibular system, such as Pilates, yoga, and Tai Chi, may also be particularly helpful. Strategies for management of large fiber neuropathies include

- Strength, gait, and balance training
- Pain management as detailed below
- Orthotics fitted with proper shoes to treat or prevent foot deformities
- Tendon lengthening for equinus caused by Achilles tendon shortening
- Bisphophonates to treat osteopenia
- Surgical reconstruction and full contact casting as necessary

Strategies for management of small fiber neuropathies include several simple measures that can protect the foot deficient in functional C-fibers from developing ulceration, and therefore, gangrene and amputation:

- Foot protection is of the utmost importance. Wearing padded socks can promote ulcer healing or reduce the likelihood of developing one [78].
- Supportive shoes with orthotics if necessary
- Regular foot and shoe inspection. Patients should inspect the plantar surface of their feet with a mirror on a daily basis. (Many are too obese to see their feet, let alone the undersurface).
- Extreme caution to prevent heat injury. Patients should test the bath water with a part of the body that is not insensate before plunging a numb foot into the water. Patients should also be cautioned against falling asleep in front of the fireplace with their insensate feet close to the fire.
- Use emollient creams to moisturize dry skin and prevent cracking and infection.

Therapies aimed at pathogenic mechanisms

Retrospective and prospective studies have suggested a relationship between hyperglycemia and the development and severity of diabetic neuropathy, and significant effects of intensive insulin treatment on prevention of neuropathy [79]. Intensive treatment of hyperglycemia in the elderly is controversial. Additionally, no epidemiologic or natural history study has defined the importance of late-onset diabetes in aged populations and IFG as risk factors for nerve function decline in very old adults. Recent data from the Cardiovascular Health Study suggest that IFG is a risk factor for autonomic neuropathy in the elderly [80].

Studies in animal models and cultured cells provide a conceptual framework for the cause and treatment of diabetic neuropathy; however, the limited translational work in diabetic patients continues to generate debate over the causes of human diabetic neuropathy, and to date we have no effective long-term treatment. Several clinical trials found that treating oxidative stress may improve peripheral and autonomic neuropathy in Type II diabetic adults [19,81–83]. Thiazolidinediones, which reduce hyperglycemia through reductions in insulin resistance and may also influence chronic inflammation, potentially impact pathways leading to peripheral neuropathy [84]. Exciting emerging evidence indicates that fibrates and statins are protective for peripheral nerve function decline in Type II diabetic adults [85]. Older adults using statins show a greater benefit than younger adults because of their higher attributable risk of cardiovascular disease [86]; however, the impact of statins on peripheral neuropathy in the elderly is not yet evaluated. A summary of the drugs that have been studied in clinical trials aimed at treating the pathogenic mechanisms of DPN is found in Table 4.

Therapy aimed at treating symptoms in patients who have sensorimotor distal polyneuropathy

It is critical to discern the underlying condition in diabetic patients who have pain. Physicians must be able to differentiate painful diabetic neuropathy from other unrelated or coexisting conditions in patients who have diabetes. The most common of these are claudication, Morton's neuroma, Charcot neuroarthropathy, fasciitis, osteoarthritis, and radiculopathy (Table 5).

Treatment strategies should aim to decrease the afferent input, reduce local inflammation, suppress sympathetic fortification of the stimulus, reduce the impact of excitatory amino acids, alter the modulation of nociceptors, and suppress Na+ channel activity (Fig. 8).

Amitriptyline is prescribed for diabetic neuropathy [87], but anticholinergic side effects such as orthostatic hypotension and possible cardiac arrhythmias [87,88] warrant caution in its use. Contraindications to amitriptyline and other tricyclic antidepressants include cardiac conduction block, long QT syndrome, myocardial infarction within 6 months, and ventricular arrhythmias or frequent premature ventricular contractions [88]. Older adults who have neuropathy are at risk for adverse events from tricyclic antidepressants, especially stability, balance, and cognitive problems [89]. For this reason, patients over 40 years old should have a screening electrocardiogram before using these medications [89].

Other commonly used drug classes include analgesics (local, simple, and narcotic), antiarrhythmics, and antiepileptic drugs (Table 6) [88]. Based on positive results from randomized, controlled trials and expert clinical opinion of members of the faculty of the Fourth International Conference on the Mechanisms and Treatment of Neuropathic Pain, recommendations for first-line medications for neuropathic pain include gabapentin, 5% lidocaine patch, opioid analgesics, tramadol hydrochloride, and tricyclic antidepressants [89]. Consideration of the safety and tolerability of different

Table 4
Treatment of diabetic neuropathy based on pathogenetic mechanisms

Abnormality	Compound	Aim of treatment	Status of RCTs
Polyol pathway ↑	Aldose reductase inhibitors	Nerve sorbitol ↓	
	Sorbinil		Withdrawn (AE)
	Tolrestat		Withdrawn (AE)
	Ponalrestat		Ineffective
	Zopolrestat		Withdrawn (marginal effects)
	Zenarestat		Withdrawn (AE)
	Lidorestat		Withdrawn (AE)
	Fidarestat		Effective in RCTs, Trials ongoing
	AS-3201		Effective in RCTs, Trials ongoing
	Epalrestat		Marketed in Japan
Myo-inositol ↓	Myo-inositol	Nerve myo-inositol ↑	Equivocal
Oxidative stress ↑	α−Lipoic acid, nutrinerve	Oxygen free radicals ↓	Effective in RCTs, trials ongoing
Nerve hypoxia ↑	Vasodilators	NBF ↑	
	ACE inhibitors		Effective in one RCT
	Prostaglandin analogs		Effective in one RCT
	phVEGF$_{165}$ gene transfer	Angiogenesis ↑	RCTs ongoing
Protein kinase C ↑	PKC β inhibitor (ruboxistaurin)	NBF ↑	Phase II +ve[a] Phase III −ve[a]
C-peptide ↓	C-peptide	NBF ↑	Studies ongoing
Neurotrophism ↓	NGF	Nerve regeneration, growth ↑	Ineffective
	BDNF	Nerve regeneration, growth ↑	Ineffective
LCFA metabolism ↓	Acetyl-L-carnitine	LCFA accumulation ↓	Ineffective
GLA synthesis ↓	γ−Linolenic acid (GLA)	EFA metabolism ↑	Withdrawn
NEG ↑	Aminoguanidine	AGE accumulation ↓	Withdrawn

Abbreviations: ACE, angiotensin-converting enzyme; AE, adverse events; AGE, advanced glycation end products; BDNF, brain-derived neurotrophic factor; EFA, essential fatty acids; GLA, gamma linolenic acid; LCFA, long-chain fatty acids; NBF, nerve blood flow; NEG, non-enzymatic glycation; NGF, nerve growth factor; PKC, protein kinase; RCTs, randomized clinical trials; ↑, increase; ↓, decrease.

[a] Casellini CM, Barlow PM, Rice AL, et al. A 6-month, randomized, double-masked, placebo-controlled study evaluating the effects of the protein kinase C-{beta} inhibitor ruboxistaurin on skin microvascular blood flow and other measures of diabetic peripheral neuropathy. Diabetes Care 2007;30:896–902.

From Boulton A, Vinik, A, Arezzo J, et al. American Diabetes Association: position statement: diabetic neuropathies. 2005.

Table 5
Common pain syndromes similar to painful diabetic neuropathy

Condition	Key characteristics and differentiating features
Claudication	Doppler ultrasonography confirms clinical diagnosis of arterial occlusion.
	Diabetic patients may present with normal extremities and absent foot pulses
	Peripheral arterial occlusion with underlying atherosclerosis
	Usually intermittent, worsened by walking; remits with rest; other signs/symptoms suggest arterial insufficiency
Morton's neuroma	Benign neuroma formation on third plantar interdigital nerve
	Generally unilateral
	More frequent in women
	Pain elicited when pressure is applied with the thumb between the first and fourth metatarsal heads
Osteoarthritis	Can be secondary to diabetes mellitus, but onset of pain is usually gradual and in one or two joints
	Differential diagnosis based on radiograph
	Morning stiffness, diminished joint motion, and flexion contractures
	Pain worsens with exercise and improves with rest.
	Radiculopathy can result.
Radiculopathy	Can be caused by diabetes, but also from arthritis or metastatic disease
	Neurologic examinations and imaging can localize lesion site
	Pain can occur in thorax, extremities, shoulder, or arm, depending on site of lesion
Charcot neuroarthropathy	May result from osteopenia caused by increased blood flow following repeated minor trauma in individuals who have diabetic neuropathy.
	Warm to hot foot with increased skin blood flow.
	Decreased warm sensory perception, vibration detection
Plantar fasciitis	Pain in plantar region of the foot
	Tenderness along plantar fascia when ankle is dorsiflexed
	Shooting or burning in the heel with each step
	Worsening pain with prolonged activity
	Often associated with calcaneal spur on radiography
Tarsal tunnel syndrome	Caused by entrapment of the posterior tibial nerve
	Pain and numbness radiate from beneath the medial malleolus to the sole.
	Clinical examination includes percussion, palpation for possible soft-tissue matter, nerve conduction studies, magnetic resonance imaging

therapies is important in avoiding adverse effects, a common result of treatment of neuropathic pain. Dosages must be titrated based on positive response, treatment adherence, and adverse events [89].

Anti-epileptic drugs (AEDs) have a long history of effectiveness in the treatment of neuropathic pain. Since 1993, nine new AEDs (felbamate, gabapentin, pregabalin, lamotrigine, topiramate, tiagabine, levetiracetam,

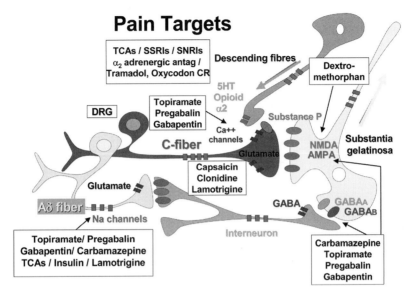

Fig. 8. Different mechanisms of pain and possible treatments: C fibers are modulated by sympathetic input with spontaneous firing of different neurotransmitters to the dorsal root ganglia, spinal cord, and cerebral cortex. Sympathetic blockers (eg, clonidine) and depletion of axonal substance P used by C fibers as their neurotransmitter (eg, by capsaicin) may improve pain. In contrast Ad fibers use Na+ channels for their conduction, and agents that inhibit Na+ exchange, such as antiepileptic drugs, tricyclic antidepressants, and insulin, may ameliorate this form of pain. Anticonvulsants (carbamazepine, gabapentin, pregabalin, topiramate) potentiate activity of g-aminobutyric acid, inhibit Na+ and Ca2+ channels, and inhibit N-methyl-D-aspartate receptors and α-amino-3-hydroxy-5-methyl-4-isoxazole propionic acid receptors. Dextromethorphan blocks N-methyl-D-aspartate receptors in the spinal cord. Tricyclic antidepressants, selective serotonin reuptake inhibitors (eg, fluoxetine), and serotonin and norepinephrine reuptake inhibitors inhibit serotonin and norepinephrine reuptake, enhancing their effect in endogenous pain-inhibitory systems in the brain. Tramadol is a central opioid analgesic. α2 antag, α2 antagonists; 5HT, 5-hydroxytryptamine; AMPA, α-amino-3-hydroxy-5-methyl-4-isoxazole propionic acid; DRG, dorsal root ganglia; GABA, g-aminobutyric acid; NMDA, N-methyl-D-aspartate; SNRIs, serotonin and norepinephrine reuptake inhibitors; SP, substance P; SSRIs, selective serotonin reuptake inhibitors; TCA, tricyclic antidepressants. (*From* Vinik A, Casellini DC, Nakave A, et al. Chapter 35. Diabetic neuropathies. 2007; with permission. Available at: http://endotext.org/diabetes/diabetes35/diabetesframe35.htm. Accessed March 10, 2008.)

oxcarbazepine, and zonisamide) have received Food and Drug Administration (FDA) approval for the adjunctive treatment of partial seizures [90] (see Table 6). Three of these drugs have also been approved for generalized seizures (felbamate, lamotrigine, topiramate) and three (felbamate, lamotrigine, oxcarbazepine) for monotherapy [90]. Principal mechanisms of action include sodium channel blockade (felbamate, lamotrigine, oxcarbazepine, topiramate, zonisamide), potentiation of gamma-aminobutyric acid (GABA) activity (tiagabine, topiramate), calcium channel blockade (felbamate, lamotrigine, topiramate, zonisamide), antagonism of glutamate at

Table 6
Drugs approved by the FDA for treatment of neuropathic pain syndrome

Medication	Indication	Beginning dosages	Titration	Maximum dosage	Duration of adequate trial
Gabapentin	Postherpetic neuralgia	100–300 mg every night or 100–300 mg three times a day	Increase by 100–300 mg three times a day every 1–7 days as tolerated	3600 mg/day (1200 mg three times a day); reduce if low creatinine clearance	3–8 weeks for titration plus 1–2 weeks at maximum tolerated dosage
Pregabaline	Postherpetic neuralgia	50 mg three times a day	Increase up to 100 mg three times a day	600 mg a day	Start with 50 mg three times a day and increase up to 100 mg three times a day over 1 week
Lamotrigine	Postherpetic neuralgia	200–400 mg every night.	Start with 25 to 50 mg every other day and increase by 25 mg every week	500 mg a day	3 to 5 weeks for titration and continue 1–2 weeks at maximum tolerated dosage
Carbamazepine[a]	Trigeminal neuralgia	200 mg/d (100 mg twice a day)	Add up to 200 mg/day in increments of 100 mg every 12 hours	1200 mg a day	
5% lidocaine patch	Postherpetic neuralgia	Maximum of three patches daily for a maximum of 12 hours	None needed	Maximum of three patches daily for a maximum of 12 hours	2 weeks
Opioid analgesics[b]	Moderate to severe pain	5–15 mg every 4 hours as needed	After 1–2 weeks, convert total daily dosage to long-acting medication as needed	No maximum with careful titration; consider evaluation by pain specialist at dosages exceeding 120–180 mg a day	4–6 weeks

Tramadol hydrochloride	Moderate to moderately severe pain	50 mg one or two times a day	Increased by 50–100 mg a day in divided doses every 3–7 days as tolerated	400 mg a day (100 mg four times a day); in patients older than 75 years, 300 mg a day in divided doses	4 weeks
Tricyclic antidepressants (eg, nortriptyline hydrochloride or desipramine hydrochloride)	Chronic pain	10–25 mg every night	Increase by 10–25 mg a day every 3–7 days as tolerated	75–150 mg a day; if blood level of active drug and its metabolite is <100 ng/mL, continue titration with caution	6–8 weeks with at least 1–2 weeks at maximum tolerated dosage
Duloxetine serotonin/ norepinephrine reuptake inhibitor	Diabetic neuropathic pain	30 mg twice a day	Increase by 60 to 60 mg twice a day. No further titration		4 weeks
Fluoxetine serotonin/ norepinephrine reuptake inhibitor	Diabetic neuropathic pain	30 mg twice a day	Increase by 60 to 60 mg twice a day. No further titration		4 weeks

[a] Tegretol prescribing information. Novartis Pharmaceuticals (East Hanover, New Jersey).

[b] Dosages given are for morphine sulfate.

Adapted from Inzitari M, Carlo A, Baldereschi M, et al. Risk and predictors of motor-performance decline in a normally functioning population-based sample of elderly subjects: the Italian Longitudinal Study on Aging. J Am Geriatr Soc 2006;54:318–24; with permission.

N-methyl-D-aspartate (NMDA) receptors (felbamate, memantine, dextrome-thorphan) or a-amino-3-hydroxy-5-methyl-4-isoxazole propionic acid (AMPA) (felbamate, topiramate), and mechanisms of action still undetermined (gabapentin, pregabalin, levetiracetam). Only two drugs have been approved by the FDA for the treatment of painful diabetic neuropathy: pregabalin and duloxetine.

Pregabalin produced significant improvements in pain scores within 1 week of treatment, which persisted for 6 to 12 weeks in four randomized controlled trials including 146 to 724 patients who had diabetic neuropathy [91–94]. Adverse events included dose-related somnolence, ataxia and confusion, peripheral edema, and constipation. A recent Canadian study evaluated the cost effectiveness of pregabalin versus gabapentin for the treatment of painful DN, concluding that pregabalin was more cost effective than gabapentin [95].

Lamotrigine (200 to 400 mg daily) is an anticonvulsant with dual-action inhibition of neuronal hyperexcitability. Two randomized, placebo-controlled studies including 720 patients showed that the drug was inconsistently effective for the treatment of pain when compared with placebo, although it was generally safe and well-tolerated [96].

In addition to providing efficacy against epilepsy, these new AEDs may also be effective in treating neuropathic pain. For example, the antiepileptic drug (AED) lamotrigine may decrease hyperexcitability in dorsal horn spinal neurons by inhibiting glutamate release-2 mechanisms and decrease spontaneous activity in regenerating primary afferent nerve fibers [97]. In addition, the "wind-up" phenomenon caused by nerve injury and the kindling that occurs in hippocampal neurons in patients who have mesial temporal sclerosis both enlist activation of NMDA receptors [98] that can be affected by felbamate [90].

The evidence supporting the use of AEDs for the treatment of PN continues to evolve. Patients who have failed one anticonvulsant may respond to another, because drugs in this class often have different mechanisms of action [89]. When these mechanisms are understood, it may prove beneficial to combine drugs for a synergistic effect. For example, a sodium channel blocker such as lamotrigine may be used with a glutamate antagonist such as felbamate. In addition, certain drugs may possess multiple mechanisms of action, which increases their likelihood of success (eg, topiramate). If pain is divided according to its derivation from different nerve fiber types (eg, Ad versus C-fiber), spinal cord or cortical, then different types of pain should respond to different therapies (Fig. 9).

Protein kinase C (PKC) activation is a critical step in the pathway to diabetic microvascular complications. It is activated by both hyperglycemia and disordered fatty-acid metabolism resulting in increased production of vasoconstrictive, angiogenic, and chemotactic cytokines, including transforming growth factor β (TGF-β), vascular endothelial growth factor (VEGF), endothelin (ET-1), and intercellular adhesion molecules (ICAMs). A multinational, randomized, phase-2, double-blind, placebo-controlled have received FDA approval for the treatment of chronic neuropathic pain syndrome [90]. Carbamazepine has FDA approval for the treatment of trigeminal neuralgia, and is effective in controlling the lightning pain of DN, and both gabapentin and lidocaine 5% patch [89] are approved for postherpetic neuralgia [89].

Special considerations

Carbamazepine, a Na+ channel blocker, is effective against trigeminal neuralgia, but is being replaced with the safer oxcarbazine, which is useful for "lightning" type pains. Lamotrigine may cause skin rashes if titrated up too rapidly, and gabapentin, whose action still remains obscure and may cause serious central nervous system (CNS) side effects, has failed in one of three studies and causes weight gain. Dextromethorphan, an NMDA receptor antagonist, was relatively weak and its successor memantine has not undergone successful trials. Topical capsaicin (three teaspoons cayenne pepper plus 1 jar cold cream) depletes substance P, but is difficult to use and can be dangerous if it contacts mucous membranes. Results from topical lidocaine or its oral equivalent mexilitine are equivocal. The anticonvulsant drug topiramate has been used successfully to treat pain in diabetic patients and also promotes weight loss and restful sleep, suggesting that the drug may have other beneficial effects apart from relieving pain [103]. Tramadol and oxycodone are weak opiods that have also shown to be effective, but require careful titration and observation.

Another type of pain, adelta pain, is described as a more deep-seated ache that does not often respond to the medications above. Several different agents have been used with varying success. Continuous intravenous insulin infusion without blood glucose lowering may be useful in these patients. The patient is admitted in the evening and usual diabetes treatment is instituted and a regular meal plan followed. NaCl is administered intravenously. In the morning, insulin is infused in a dose of 0.8 to 1.0 units hourly. Pain reduction usually occurs within 48 hours, at which time the insulin infusion is discontinued. If this measure fails, there are several medications available that may abolish the pain.

Summary

Diabetic neuropathy is a heterogeneous disease with diverse pathology. Recognition of the clinical homologue of these pathologic processes is the first step in achieving the appropriate form of intervention. Treatment should be individualized such that the particular manifestation and underlying pathogenesis of each patient's unique clinical presentation is considered. In older adults, special care should be taken to manage pain while optimizing daily function and mobility, with the fewest adverse side effects from medication. Older adults are at great risk for falling

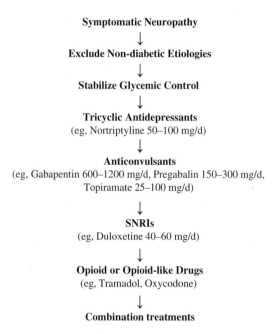

Fig. 9. Algorithm for the management of symptomatic diabetic neuropathy: Nonpharm
logic, topical, or physical therapies can be useful at any time (capsaicin, acupuncture,
The only two drugs approved by in the United States for the treatment of painful diabetic
ropathy are pregabalin and duloxetine; however, based on the number needed to treat (N
tricyclic antidepressants are the most cost-effective ones. (*From* Vinik A, Casellini DC, Na
A, et al. Chapter 35. Diabetic neuropathies. 2007; with permission. Available at: http://endo
org/diabetes/diabetes35/diabetesframe35.htm. Accessed March 10, 2008.)

trial with ruboxistaurin (a PKC-β inhibitor) failed to achieve the prim
end points, although significant changes were observed in a number
domains [99]. Nevertheless, in a subgroup of patients who had less sev
DN (sural nerve action potential greater than 0.5 μV) at baseline a
clinically significant symptoms, a statistically significant improvement
symptoms and vibratory detection thresholds was observed in the rubox
taurin-treated groups as compared with placebo [100]. A smaller, sing
center study recently published showed improvement in symptom scor
endothelium-dependent skin blood flow measurements, and quality of l
scores in the ruboxistaurin treated group [101]. These studies and t
NATHAN studies have pointed out the change in natural history of D
with the advent of therapeutic lifestyle change, statins, and angiotensi
converting enzyme (ACE) inhibitors, which have slowed the progressic
of DN and drastically changed the requirements for placebo-controlle
studies [102].

Although it would be preferable to rely on FDA-approved medicatior
for the treatment of DN, no drugs have yet received an indication for th
purpose. As shown in Table 6, only a few drugs, including two AED

and fractures because of instability and weakness, and require strength exercises and coordination training. Ultimately, agents that address large fiber dysfunction will be essential if we are to reduce the gross impairment of QOL and ADLs that neuropathy visits upon the older person who has diabetes.

References

[1] Vinik AI, Mitchell BD, Leichter SB, et al. Epidemiology of the complications of diabetes. In: Leslie RDG, Robbins DC, editors. Diabetes: clinical science in practice. Cambridge (United Kingdom): Cambridge University Press; 1995. p. 221–87.

[2] Knuiman M, Welborn T, McCann V, et al. Prevalence of diabetic complications in relation to risk factors. Diabetes 1986;35:1332–9.

[3] Young MJ, Boulton AJM, MacLeod AF, et al. A multicenter study of the prevalence of diabetic peripheral neuropathy in the United Kingdom hospital clinic population. Diabetologia 1993;36:1–5.

[4] Holzer SE, Camerota A, Martens L, et al. Costs and duration of care for lower extremity ulcers in patients with diabetes. Clin Ther 1998;20:169–81.

[5] Caputo GM, Cavanagh PR, Ulbrecht JS, et al. Assessment and management of foot disease in patients with diabetes. N Engl J Med 1994;331:854–60.

[6] Menz HB, Lord SR, St George R, et al. Walking stability and sensorimotor function in older people with diabetic peripheral neuropathy. Arch Phys Med Rehabil 2004;85: 245–52.

[7] Maty SC, Fried LP, Volpato S, et al. Patterns of disability related to diabetes mellitus in older women. J Gerontol A Biol Sci Med Sci 2004;59:148–53.

[8] Richardson JK, Thies SB, DeMott TK, et al. A comparison of gait characteristics between older women with and without peripheral neuropathy in standard and challenging environments. J Am Geriatr Soc 2004;52:1532–7.

[9] Gregg EW, Sorlie P, Paulose-Ram R, et al. Prevalence of lower-extremity disease in the US adult population 40 years of age with and without diabetes: 1999–2000 National Health and Nutrition Examination Survey. Diabetes Care 2004;27:1591–7.

[10] Vinik AI, Erbas T. Recognizing and treating diabetic autonomic neuropathy. Cleve Clin J Med 2001;68(11):928–44.

[11] Vinik A, Mehrabyan A. Diagnosis and management of diabetic autonomic neuropathy. Compr Ther 2003;29(2/3):130–45.

[12] Lindenlaub T, Sommer C. Cytokines in sural nerve biopsies from inflammatory and non-inflammatory neuropathies. Acta Neuropathol 2003;105:593–602.

[13] Jude EB, Abbott CA, Young MJ, et al. The potential role of cell adhesion molecules in the pathogens of diabetic neuropathy. Diabetologia 1998;41:330–6.

[14] Brownlee M. Advanced products of nonenzymatic glycosylation and the pathogenesis of diabetic complications. In: Rifkin H, Porte D, editors. Diabetes mellitus: theory and practice. 1st edition. New York: Elsevier; 1990. p. 229–45.

[15] Laghi PF, Pastorelli M, Beermann U, et al. Peripheral neuropathy associated with ischemic vascular disease of the lower limbs. Angiology 1996;47:569–77.

[16] Young MJ, Veves A, Smith JV, et al. Restoring lower limb blood flow improves conduction velocity in diabetic patients. Diabetologia 1995;38:1051–4.

[17] Liu B, Gao HM, Wang JY, et al. Role of nitric oxide in inflammation-mediated neurodegeneration. Ann NY Acad Sci 2002;962:318–31.

[18] Pop-Busui R, Sima A, Stevens M. Diabetic neuropathy and oxidative stress. Diabetes Metab Res Rev 2006;22:257–73.

[19] Ziegler D, Hanefeld M, Ruhnau KJ, et al. Treatment of symptomatic diabetic polyneuropathy with the antioxidant alpha-lipoic acid: a 7-month multicenter randomized controlled

trial (ALADIN III Study). ALADIN III Study Group. Alpha-Lipoic Acid in Diabetic Neuropathy. Diabetes Care 1999;22:1296–301.

[20] Bruunsgaard H, Pedersen M, Pedersen BK. Aging and proinflammatory cytokines. Curr Opin Hematol 2001;8:131–6.

[21] Yudkin JS, Stehouwer CD, Emeis JJ, et al. C-reactive protein in healthy subjects: associations with obesity, insulin resistance, and endothelial dysfunction: a potential role for cytokines originating from adipose tissue? Arterioscler Thromb Vasc Biol 1999;19: 972–8.

[22] Ford ES. Body mass index, diabetes, and C-reactive protein among U.S. adults. Diabetes Care 1999;22:1971–7.

[23] Festa A, D'Agostino R Jr, Howard G, et al. Chronic subclinical inflammation as part of the insulin resistance syndrome: the Insulin Resistance Atherosclerosis Study (IRAS). Circulation 2000;102:42–7.

[24] Frohlich M, Imhof A, Berg G, et al. Association between C-reactive protein and features of the metabolic syndrome: a population-based study. Diabetes Care 2000;23:1835–9.

[25] Temelkova-Kurktschiev T, Siegert G, Bergmann S, et al. Subclinical inflammation is strongly related to insulin resistance but not to impaired insulin secretion in a high risk population for diabetes. Metabolism 2002;51:743–9.

[26] Vinik A, Mehrabyan A, Colen L, et al. Focal entrapment neuropathies in diabetes. Diabetes Care 2004;27:1783–8.

[27] Wilbourn AJ. Diabetic entrapment and compression neuropathies. In: Dyck PJ, Thomas PK, editors. Diabetic neuropathy. Philadelphia: Saunders; 1999. p. 481–508.

[28] Kapritskaya Y, Novak C, Mackinnon S. Prevalence of smoking, obesity, diabetes mellitus and thyroid disease in patients with carpal tunnel syndrome. Ann Plast Surg 2002;48(3): 269–79.

[29] Vinik AI, Holland MT, LeBeau JM, et al. Diabetic neuropathies. Diabetes Care 1992;15: 1926–75.

[30] Leedman PJ, Davis S, Harrison LC. Diabetic amyotrophy. Reassessment of the clinical spectrum. Aust NZJ Med 1988;18:768–73.

[31] Barohn RJ, Sahenk Z, Warmolts JR, et al. The Bruns-Garland syndrome (diabetic amyotrophy). Arch Neurol 1991;48:1130–5.

[32] Diabetes Control and Complications Trial Research Group. Effect of intensive diabetes treatment on nerve conduction in the Diabetes Control And Complications Trial. Ann Internal Med 1995;122:561–8.

[33] The effect of intensive treatment of diabetes on the development and progression of long-term complications in insulin-dependent diabetes mellitus. Diabetes Control and Complications Trial Research Group. N Engl J Med 1993;329:977–86.

[34] Vinik AI, Pittenger GL, Milicevic Z, et al. Autoimmune mechanisms in the pathogenesis of diabetic neuropathy. In: Eisenbarth RG, editor. Molecular mechanisms of endocrine and organ specific autoimmunity. 1st edition. Georgetown, TX: Landes Company; 1998. p. 217–51.

[35] Steck AJ, Kappos L. Gangliosides and autoimmune neuropathies: classification and clinical aspects of autoimmune neuropathies. J Neurol Neurosurg Psychiatry 1994;(57 Suppl): 26–8.

[36] Vinik A. Diagnosis and management of diabetic neuropathy. Clin Geriatr Med 1999;15: 293–319.

[37] Milicevic Z, Pittenger GL, Stansberry KB, et al. Raised anti-ganglioside GM1 antibody (GM1 Ab) titers in a subset of patients with distal symmetric polyneuropathy (DSPN) [abstract]. Diabetes 1997;46:125A.

[38] Sharma K, Cross J, Farronay O, et al. Demyelinating neuropathy in diabetes mellitus. Arch Neurol 2002;59:758–65.

[39] Krendel DA, Costigan DA, Hopkins LC. Successful treatment of neuropathies in patients with diabetes mellitus. Arch Neurol 1995;52:1053–61.

[40] Barney Y, Bossmeyer R, Kokomen E. Neurological manifestations of aging. Am Ger Soc 1990;32:411–9.

[41] Maki BE, Holliday PJ, Fernie GR. Aging and postural control. A comparison of spontaneous- and induced-sway balance tests. J Am Geriatr Soc 1990;38:1–9.

[42] Potvin AR, Syndulko K, Tourtellotte WW, et al. Human neurologic function and the aging process. J Am Geriatr Soc 1980;1:1–9.

[43] Vinik AI, Suwanwalaikorn S, Stansberry KB, et al. Quantitative measurement of cutaneous perception in diabetic neuropathy. Muscle Nerve 1995;18:574–84.

[44] Yu RK, Ariga T, Kohriyama T, et al. Autoimmune mechanisms in peripheral neuropathies. Ann Neurol 1990;27(Suppl 1):S30–5.

[45] Evans W. Functional and metabolic consequences of sarcopenia. J Nutr 1997;127: 998S–1003S.

[46] Baumgartner RN. Body composition in healthy aging. Ann N Y Acad Sci 2000;904:437–48.

[47] Andersen JL. Muscle fibre type adaptation in the elderly human muscle. Scand J Med Sci Sports 2003;13:40–7.

[48] Bus SA, Yang QX, Wang JH, et al. Intrinsic muscle atrophy and toe deformity in the diabetic neuropathic foot. Diabetes Care 2002;25:1444–50.

[49] Andersen H, Gjerstad MD, Jakobsen J. Atrophy of foot muscles: a measure of diabetic neuropathy. Diabetes Care 2004;27:2382–5.

[50] Vinik EJ, Hayes RP, Oglesby A, et al. The development and validation of the Norfolk QOL-DN, a new measure of patients' perception of the effects of diabetes and diabetic neuropathy. Diabetes Technol Ther 2005;7:497–508.

[51] Resnick HE, Stansberry KB, Harris TB, et al. Diabetes, peripheral neuropathy, and old age disability. Muscle Nerve 2002;25:43–50.

[52] Strotmeyer ES, Cauley JA, Schwartz AV, et al. Reduced peripheral nerve function is related to lower hip BMD and calcaneal QUS in older white and black adults: the health, aging, and body composition study. J Bone Miner Res 2006;21:1803–10.

[53] Lauretani F. Axonal degeneration affects muscle density in older men and women. Neurobiol Aging 2006;27:1145–54.

[54] Inzitari M, Carlo A, Baldereschi M, et al. Risk and predictors of motor-performance decline in a normally functioning population-based sample of elderly subjects: the Italian Longitudinal Study on Aging. J Am Geriatr Soc 2006;54:318–24.

[55] Koski K, Luukinen H, Laippala P, et al. Risk factors for major injurious falls among the home-dwelling elderly by functional abilities. A prospective population-based study. Gerontology 1998;44:232–8.

[56] Schwartz AV, Hillier TA, Sellmeyer DE, et al. Older women with diabetes have a higher risk of falls: a prospective study. Diabetes Care 2002;25:1749–54.

[57] Zhuang HX, Snyder CK, Pu SF, et al. Insulin-like growth factors reverse or arrest diabetic neuropathy: effects on hyperalgesia and impaired nerve regeneration in rats. Exp Neurol 1996;140:198–205.

[58] Said G, Goulon-Goreau C, Lacroix C, et al. Nerve biopsy findings in different patterns of proximal diabetic neuropathy. Ann Neurol 1994;35:559–69.

[59] Young MJ, Marshall M, Adams JE, et al. Osteopenia, neurological dysfunction, and the development of Charcot neuroarthropathy. Diabetes Care 1995;18:34–8.

[60] Haslbeck KM, Bierhaus A, Erwin S, et al. Receptor for advanced glycation endproduct (RAGE)-mediated nuclear factor-kappaB activation in vasculitic neuropathy. Muscle Nerve 2004;29:853–60.

[61] Grant WP, Sullivan R, Sonenshine DE, et al. Electron microscopic investigation of the effects of diabetes mellitus on the Achilles tendon. J Foot Ankle Surg 1997;36:272–8.

[62] Anderson JJ, Woelffer KE, Holtzman JJ, et al. Bisphosphonates for the treatment of Charcot neuroarthropathy. J Foot Ankle Surg 2004;43:285–9.

[63] Baik HW, Russell RM. Vitamin B12 deficiency in the elderly. Annu Rev Nutr 1999;19: 357–77.

[64] Stone KL, Bauer DC, Sellmeyer D, et al. Low serum vitamin B-12 levels are associated with increased hip bone loss in older women: a prospective study. J Clin Endocrinol Metab 2004; 89:1217–21.

[65] Dhonukshe-Rutten RA, Pluijm SM, de Groot LC, et al. Homocysteine and vitamin B12 status relate to bone turnover markers, broadband ultrasound attenuation, and fractures in healthy elderly people. J Bone Miner Res 2005;20:921–9.

[66] Tucker KL. Low plasma vitamin B12 is associated with lower BMD: the Framingham Osteoporosis Study. J Bone Miner Res 2005;20:152–8.

[67] Eussen SJ, de Groot LC, Clarke R, et al. Oral cyanocobalamin supplementation in older people with vitamin B12 deficiency: a dose-finding trial. Arch Intern Med 2005;165: 1167–72.

[68] Newman AB, Siscovick DS, Manolio TA, et al. Ankle-arm index as a marker of atherosclerosis in the Cardiovascular Health Study. Cardiovascular Health Study (CHS) Collaborative Research Group. Circulation 1993;88:837–45.

[69] McDermott MM, Guralnik JM, Albay M, et al. Impairments of muscles and nerves associated with peripheral arterial disease and their relationship with lower extremity functioning: the InCHIANTI Study. J Am Geriatr Soc 2004;52:405–10.

[70] Hirsch AT, Criqui MH, Treat-Jacobson D, et al. Peripheral arterial disease detection, awareness, and treatment in primary care. JAMA 2001;286:1317–24.

[71] Hankey GJ, Norman PE, Eikelboom JW. Medical treatment of peripheral arterial disease. JAMA 2006;295:547–53.

[72] Ford ES, Giles WH, Dietz WH. Prevalence of the metabolic syndrome among US adults: findings from the third National Health and Nutrition Examination Survey. JAMA 2002; 287(3):356–9.

[73] Costa LA, Canani LH, Lisboa HR, et al. Aggregation of features of the metabolic syndrome is associated with increased prevalence of chronic complications in type 2 diabetes. Diabet Med 2004;21:252–5.

[74] Isomaa B, Henricsson M, Almgren P, et al. The metabolic syndrome influences the risk of chronic complications in patients with Type II diabetes. Diabeologia 2001;44:1148–54.

[75] Cavanagh PR, Derr JA, Ulbrecht JS, et al. Problems with gait and posture in neuropathic patients with insulin-dependent diabetes mellitus. Diabet Med 1992;9:469–74.

[76] Nelson ME, Fiatarone MA, Morganti CM, et al. Effects of high-intensity strength training on multiple risk factors for osteoporotic fractures. A randomized controlled trial. JAMA 1994;272:1909–14.

[77] Liu-Ambrose T, Khan KM, Eng JJ, et al. Resistance and agility training reduce fall risk in women aged 75 to 85 with low bone mass: a 6-month randomized, controlled trial. J Am Geriatr Soc 2004;52:657–65.

[78] Murray H, Veves A, Young M, et al. Role of experimental socks in the care of the high risk diabetic foot. A multi-center patient evaluation study. American group for the study of experimental hosiery in the diabetic foot. Diabetes Care 1993;16:1190–2.

[79] Pirart J. Diabetes mellitus and its degenerative complications: a prospective study of 4400 patients observed between 1947 and 1973. Diabetes Care 1978;1:252–63.

[80] Stein PK, Barzilay JI, Domitrovich PP, et al. The relationship of heart rate and heart rate variability to non-diabetic fasting glucose levels and the metabolic syndrome: the Cardiovascular Health Study. Diabet Med 2007;24:855–63.

[81] Ziegler D, Schatz H, Conrad F, et al. Effects of treatment with the antioxidant alpha-lipoic acid on cardiac autonomic neuropathy in NIDDM patients. A 4-month randomized controlled multicenter trial (DEKAN Study). Deutsche Kardiale Autonome Neuropathie. Diabetes Care 1997;20:369–73.

[82] Ruhnau KJ, Meissner HP, Finn R, et al. Effects of 3-week oral treatment with the antioxidant thioctic acid (alpha-lipoic acid) in symptomatic diabetic polyneuropathy. Diabet Med 1999;16(12):1040–3.

[83] Valensi P, Le DC, Richard JL, et al. A multicenter, double-blind, safety study of QR-333 for the treatment of symptomatic diabetic peripheral neuropathy. A preliminary report. J Diabetes Complications 2005;19:247–53.

[84] Viberti G. Thiazolidinediones-benefits on microvascular complications of type 2 diabetes. J Diabetes Complications 2005;19:168–77.

[85] Davis T, Yeap B, Bruce D, et al. Lipid-lowering therapy protects against peripheral sensory neuropathy in type 2 diabetes. Diabetes 2007.

[86] Jacobson TA. Overcoming "ageism" bias in the treatment of hypercholesterolaemia: a review of safety issues with statins in the elderly. Drug Saf 2006;29:421–48.

[87] Coppini DV, Young PJ, Weng C, et al. Outcome on diabetic foot complications in relation to clinical examination and quantitative sensory testing: a case-control study. Diabet Med 1998;15:765–71.

[88] Morello CM, Leckband SG, Stoner CP, et al. Randomized double-blind study comparing the efficacy of gabapentin with amitriptyline on diabetic peripheral neuropathy pain. Arch Intern Med 1999;159:1931–7.

[89] Dworkin RH, Backonja M, Rowbotham MC, et al. Advances in neuropathic pain: diagnosis, mechanisms, and treatment recommendations. Arch Neurol 2003;60:1524–34.

[90] LaRoche SM, Helmers SL. The new antiepileptic drugs: scientific review. JAMA 2004;291:605–14.

[91] Rosenstock J, Tuchman M, LaMoreaux L, et al. Pregabalin for the treatment of painful diabetic peripheral neuropathy: a double-blind, placebo-controlled trial. Pain 2004;110:628–38.

[92] Freynhagen R, Strojek K, Griesing T, et al. Efficacy of pregabalin in neuropathic pain evaluated in a 12-week, randomised, double-blind, multicentre, placebo-controlled trial of flexible- and fixed-dose regimens. Pain 2005;115:254–63.

[93] Richter RW, Portenoy R, Sharma U, et al. Relief of painful diabetic peripheral neuropathy with pregabalin: a randomized, placebo-controlled trial. J Pain 2005;6:253–60.

[94] Frampton JE, Scott LJ. Pregabalin: in the treatment of painful diabetic peripheral neuropathy. Drugs 2004;64:2813–20.

[95] Tarride JE, Gordon A, Vera-Llonch M, et al. Cost-effectiveness of pregabalin for the management of neuropathic pain associated with diabetic peripheral neuropathy and postherpetic neuralgia: a Canadian perspective. Clin Ther 2006;28:1922–34.

[96] Vinik AI, Tuchman M, Safirstein B, et al. Lamotrigine for treatment of pain associated with diabetic neuropathy: results of two randomized, double-blind, placebo-controlled studies. Pain 2007;128:169–79.

[97] Eisenberg E, Lurie Y, Braker C, et al. Lamotrigine reduces painful diabetic neuropathy: a randomized, controlled study. Neurology 2001;57:505–9.

[98] Backonja MM. Use of anticonvulsants for treatment of neuropathic pain. Neurology 2002;59:S14–7.

[99] Vinik A, Bril V, Kempler P, et al. Treatment of symptomatic diabetic peripheral neuropathy with protein kinase CB inhibitor ruboxistaurin mesylate during a 1-year randomized, placebo-controlled, double-blind clinical trial. Clin Ther 2005;27:1164S–80S.

[100] Vinik AI, Bril V, Litchy WJ, et al. Sural sensory action potential identifies diabetic peripheral neuropathy responders to therapy. Muscle Nerve 2005;32:619–25.

[101] Casellini CM, Barlow PM, Rice AL, et al. A 6-month, randomized, double-masked, placebo-controlled study evaluating the effects of the protein kinase C-{beta} inhibitor ruboxistaurin on skin microvascular blood flow and other measures of diabetic peripheral neuropathy. Diabetes Care 2007;30:896–902.

[102] Ziegler D, Low P, Samigullin R, et al. Effect of 4-year antioxident treatment with alpha-lipoic acid in diabetic polyneuropathy. The NATHAN Trail. Diabetes 2007;56:A2.

[103] Raskin P, Donofrio P, Rosenthal N, et al. Topiramate vs placebo in painful diabetic neuropathy: analgesic and metabolic effects. Neurology 2004;63:865–73.

ELSEVIER
SAUNDERS

CLINICS IN
GERIATRIC
MEDICINE

Clin Geriatr Med 24 (2008) 437–454

Insulin Resistance Syndrome and Glucose Dysregulation in the Elderly

Angela D. Mazza, DO*

Division of Endocrinology, Saint Louis University, 1042 South Grand Boulevard, St. Louis, MO 63104, USA

"Syndrome" is a frequently used term of Greek derivation that literally means "runs together." In medicine it usually is used to refer to a grouping of clinically recognizable features that may or may not have an elucidated underlying disease state. Accordingly, the term "insulin resistance syndrome," also known as "metabolic syndrome," is a grouping of clinically identifiable factors, including insulin resistance, dyslipidemia, and hypertension. Although each feature is risk factor for disease on its own, together they increase the probability of complications, morbidity, and mortality of further disease states of type 2 diabetes mellitus and cardiovascular disease. Conflicting evidence exists as to whether metabolic syndrome itself may predict cardiovascular risk more strongly than its individual components. Nonetheless, metabolic syndrome is associated with increased risk of coronary disease not entirely accounted for by traditional risk factors. This finding supports an association with more nontraditional atherogenic etiologies leading back to insulin resistance, such as small, dense low-density lipoprotein (LDL), triglyceride-rich lipoprotein, and low-grade inflammation with a propensity for a prothrombotic state. Metabolic syndrome is associated with an increased risk of developing cardiovascular disease with or without pre-existing diabetes. The presence of metabolic syndrome in individuals who do not have diabetes markedly increases the chance of developing type 2 diabetes. Current guidelines for metabolic syndrome focus primarily on long-term reduction of the risk of diabetes and of cardiovascular disease.

* Division of Endocrinology and Metabolism, Department of Internal Medicine, Saint Louis University Health Sciences Center, 1320 South Grand Boulevard, Saint Louis, MO 63104.

E-mail address: amazza1@slu.edu

0749-0690/08/$ - see front matter © 2008 Elsevier Inc. All rights reserved.
doi:10.1016/j.cger.2008.03.006   *geriatric.theclinics.com*

Epidemiology of insulin resistance

The prevalence of diabetes in the general population is growing at a rate that is commonly referred to epidemic in proportions, caused largely by the rise of obesity and by lifestyle changes. Twenty million individuals have diabetes, and an additional 26% of the population in the United States has impaired fasting glucose levels. The core element of insulin resistance, however, is the hyperglycemic development of diabetes that increases with advancing age [1]. Therefore, as the aging population continues to grow and the average life expectancy increases, so does the appearance of glucose dysregulation and resulting diabetes. Currently, about 20% of patients over 65 years of age suffer from diabetes.

Diabetes is a complex chronic illness affecting most races and generations. On the basis of morbidity, mortality, and cost, it is a disease state that constitutes a substantial health burden [2]. Diabetes can be difficult to treat in the general patient, and older patients present additional challenges. The Third National Health and Nutrition Examination Survey conducted from 1988 to 1994 (NHANES III) showed that the prevalence of diabetes increases significantly with age as well as being higher among certain racial minority populations. Accordingly, the health care use, including office and inpatient visits, attributed to diabetes in an older population was substantial [3,4]. NHANES 1999–2000 followed up to demonstrate that uncontrolled blood pressure and cholesterol and a rise in the prevalence of type 2 diabetes at an earlier age result in time-dependent vascular complications. Patients who have diabetes are at increased risk for vascular macrovascular disease (coronary artery disease and stroke) and microvascular disease (retinopathy, neuropathy, nephropathy). Improved glycemic control reduces or prevents these complications.

Etiology and pathophysiology of insulin resistance

Insulin resistance syndrome has been the subject of a great amount of research in recent years. Recognition of a "hypertriglyceridemia" syndrome can be dated back to the mid-sixteenth century, and its association with increased visceral obesity and elevated blood pressure was recognized in the following century. In the 1980s the term "syndrome X" was coined by Reaven [5] to designate a grouping of these risk factors. Although type 1 diabetes mellitus is the result of pancreatic destruction, type 2 diabetes results from a progressive disease state and decompensation. Insulin resistance was seen to be common both in patients who had type 2 diabetes and in patients who had impaired glucose tolerance, as a result of the pancreatic β cell's attempt to maintain glucose homeostasis in the face of chronic hyperglycemia and increased free fatty acids. The production of tumor necrosis factor alpha and other cytokines from adipocytes has been correlated with the development of diabetes and insulin resistance through the induction nitric oxide synthase. Insulin sensitizers, such as metformin and the thiazolidinediones, have been shown to inhibit this nitric oxide synthase activity.

Increased LDL, decreased high-density lipoprotein (HDL), and hypertension were noted to be concomitant variables that may be present in one individual and may be very important to the development of both diabetes and cardiovascular disease in that person [6–9]. Clinical criteria for these components of high-risk state established by the third report of the National Cholesterol Education Program's Adult Treatment Panel (NCEP-ATP III), the World Health Organization, and the International Diabetes Foundation (IDF) are listed in Table 1 [5,10,11]. The ambiguity of these criteria has led to debate; in practice, all cardiovascular risk factors should treated by clinicians without "syndrome" qualification [12]. A recent large Danish population-based study comparing both the IDF and NCEP criteria in about 2500 patients without major cardiovascular disease at baseline found insulin resistance to be an independent risk factor of heart disease, although to date no large, randomized study has demonstrated that reduction of insulin resistance improves cardiovascular outcome [13]. Low heart rate recovery at exercise test is an additional predictor of cardiovascular morbidity and mortality that, in a recent cross-sectional study of 75-year-old free-living participants, was found to be associated strongly with the components of metabolic syndrome, according to NCEP criteria

Table 1

International Diabetes Foundation, National Cholesterol Education Program, and World Health Organization definitions of metabolic syndrome

International Diabetes Foundation definition	NCEP definition	WHO definition
Central obesity (waist circumference)	At least three of following: Fasting glucose	Hyperinsulinemia or fasting plasma glucose ≥ 110 mg/dL
>94 cm in white men	≥110 mg/dL	And at least two of the following:
>90 cm in Asian men	Abdominal obesity with	Abdominal obesity with waist:
>80 cm in women	waist circumference:	hip ratio:
Plus any two	>102 cm in men	>0.9 in men
of the following:	>88 cm in women	>0.85 in women
Triglycerides > 1.7 nmol/L	Serum triglycerides	Dyslipidemia:
(150 mg/dL)	≥ 150 g/dL	Serum triglycerides
Reduced HDL:	Serum HDL < 40 mg/dL	≥ 150 mg/dL or HDL
<1.08 nmol/L (40 mg/dL)	Blood pressure	cholesterol < 35 mg/dL
in males	≥ 130/85 mm Hg	Blood pressure
<1.22 nmol/L (50mg/dL)		≥ 140/90 mm Hg
in females		
Raised blood pressure:		
>130 mm Hg systolic or		
>85 mm Hg diastolic		
Raised fasting blood glucose		
> 5.6 nmol/L (100 mg/dL)		

Abbreviation: HDL, high-density lipoprotein.

[14]. The syndrome of geriatric frailty has been associated with features of metabolic syndrome; however, in a recent analysis using physiologic determinants, such as insulin resistance as measured by homeostasis model assessment score (IR-HOMA), increased inflammation, coagulation factor levels, and elevated blood pressure, only IR-HOMA and inflammation were associated with increased incidence of frailty; insulin resistance was the component more largely associated with a generalized decline [15]. In the general population, additional psychosocial factors including depression and anxiety, inadequate emotional support, and negative life events (which vary by race and gender) are associated with metabolic dysregulation. In the geriatric population, a strong association can be seen with overall lack of emotional support coupled with negative past life events, so these psychosocial risk factors might represent targets that could be recognized on patient evaluation and influenced by patient management. The association with depressive or anxiety symptoms is not as strong [16].

Diabetes in its essence is a metabolic disorder. Although type 1 diabetes is thought to be autoimmune in nature, characterized by a decreased or lack of insulin secretion, and usually is seen in younger people, type 2 diabetes is associated with age and obesity (Fig. 1). Most patients seem to have a genetic

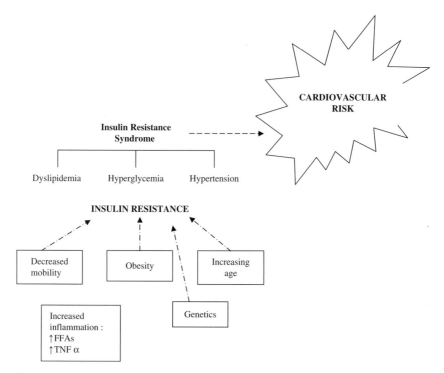

Fig. 1. Insulin resistance syndrome in the geriatric population is influenced multifactorially and constitutes a cardiovascular risk. FFAs, free fatty acids; TNFa, tumor necrosis factor-α.

risk as well that unveils an existing defect in insulin secretion [17]. There are additional environmental factors that interact with genetic susceptibility in the pathogenesis of type 2 diabetes. These factors are associated with pre-existing obesity, including an elevation in free fatty acids (as stated previously), increased release of tumor necrosis factor-α, increased synthesis of interleukin-1-β by β cells, a deficiency of adiponectin, and a multitude of other factors in the milieu [18,19].

Insulin resistance seems to be associated with increased age, as demonstrated by numerous population studies [20]. The exact age-associated mechanism is unclear, although defects in mitochondrial oxidative and phosphorylation may have an influence. In comparison with lean young controls, elderly subjects matched for properties including lean body mass and fat mass had higher circulating insulin concentrations and higher levels of basal glucose and free fatty acids during glucose challenge and also had increased intramyocellular and liver fat levels by magnetic resonance spectroscopy (MRS). Both mitochondrial oxidative activity and phosphorylation activity were decreased by about 40%, supporting an association with aging and related insulin resistance [21].

Hyperglycemia has been associated with inflammation in general. A connection has been established among diabetes, inflammation, and disability in older persons. Uncertainty exists to whether inflammation and obesity cause a decline in functional status or if disability is a result of diabetes itself. A recent study of the inflammatory markers C-reactive protein and interleukin-6 in adults considered to be well functioning suggested that increased inflammation correlated negatively with persistent functional limitation [22].

Insulin resistance and obesity

Key to the understanding of insulin resistance and the development of overt diabetes is the eventual time course of insulin resistance associated with obesity. This association is seen in modern Western society, where food intake for many individuals is excessive, and also, strikingly can be observed in animal studies in the wild. A study looking at the effects of an abundant, calorie-rich food supply on wild baboons found that a metabolic-like syndrome evolved, as evidenced by comparative increases in glucose, insulin, and lipid levels [23].

The evaluation of actual body fat distribution is helpful in evaluating the level of insulin sensitivity. Studies using proton MRS for noninvasive quantifications of nonfat tissues, including muscle and liver, have shown this modality can provide further insight. In the muscle, MRS can differentiate between extramyocellular and intramyocellular lipid and, in euglycemic-hyperinsulinemia clamp conditions, shows that fat infiltration in muscle fibers correlates with decreased insulin sensitivity [24]. Furthermore, MRS demonstrates that higher liver fat correlates with lower insulin sensitivity, adding to existing knowledge about the importance of insulin sensitivity in suppressing endogenous hepatic glucose production [25].

Insulin resistance and the adipocyte

A field of research that is adding to the current understanding of the biochemical aspects of insulin resistance is the study of adipocytes. An adipocyte is a specialized cell that is able to store excess energy in the form of lipids and has an almost unlimited capacity for growth in accordance with metabolic needs. The adipocyte has numerous types of receptors, including receptors for traditional endocrine hormones, such as insulin, glucagon, and thyroid-stimulating hormone, and for nuclear hormone receptors, cytokine receptors, and catecholamine receptors, which allow adipose tissue to receive both central and peripheral signaling [26]. In response, adipocytes can produces adipocyte-specific proteins known as "adipokines" that have been found to have local and systemic effects important to glucose homeostasis.

Adiponectin is an adipokine that has been the focus of many studies in recent years. An inverse association exists between adiponectin and insulin resistance. Adiponectin enhances insulin-mediated repression of glucose production in the liver. In vitro research using primary hepatocytes exposed to differing levels of insulin in adiponectin presence or absence show that adiponectin enhances even very small amounts of insulin significantly [27]. Other than weight loss, the only approach currently shown to improve adiponectin levels significantly is the use of activators of peroxisome proliferator-activated receptor-γ (PPAR-γ) [28], which is discussed later in this article.

Current and prospective therapies for insulin resistance syndrome

Because type 2 diabetes is a disease with such a serious and expensive course, especially in the older population, the best treatment is the prevention of metabolic dysregulation to this point. One of the strongest and most highly studied interventions to date is lifestyle modification. The Diabetes Prevention Program Research Group investigated, on a large, randomized scale, the effects of lifestyle modifications, medical treatment with metformin, and placebo in the development of diabetes in high-risk individuals. (In a later study, more than half of the population was determined actually to have metabolic syndrome Ref. [29].) Although both lifestyle changes and biguanide therapy deterred or prevented diabetes in the overall studied population, modifications in lifestyle most strongly influenced patients older than 60 years of age [30]. The importance of lifestyle modifications in this study reflected prior findings in Finland and China [31,32].

Medical nutrition therapy

Therapeutic management of insulin resistance in the general population usually focuses first on lifestyle modification in the form of medical nutrition therapy. Medical nutrition therapy consists of adequate macro- and micro-nutrient intake in addition to weight management, usually through decreased intake and increased energy expenditure [32,33]. These principles are less straightforward in the elderly population. Dietary restriction and weight loss are not recommended, because the results can lead to increased frailty and inadequate micronutrient intake [33–35]. Increasing frailty is associated independently with an increased risk of falling and fracture and subsequent overall mortality [36]. In addition, studies in the long-term care setting have failed to demonstrate the utility of dietary intervention to control diabetes [37,38]. A single study demonstrated increased mortality in older persons who had hyperglycemia and who lost weight [39]. Further-more, the American Diabetes Association guidelines do not recommend a therapeutic diet in nursing home residents who have diabetes in [40].

Omega-3 polyunsaturated fatty acids (PUFAs) are a group of polyunsat-urated fats that can be found in fish sources in the form of eicosapentaenoic acid and docosahexaenoic acid and in some vegetables, oils, and nuts in the form of a alpha-linolenic acid [41]. Several studies have evaluated the ben-eficial impact of PUFAs in fish oil in the secondary prevention of cardiovas-cular end points. The Gruppo Italiano per lo Studio della Sopravvivenza nell'Infarto Miocardico study supported the possibility of an anti-arrhyth-mic effect in addition to a significant reduction in mortality early in the course of treatment with PUFAs in survivors of recent myocardial infarc-tion [42]. A separate study found a strong association with reduced risk of sudden death in apparently healthy patients [43]. Three to 12 g of PUFAs daily have been shown to decrease triglycerides when used in adjunct to diet in patients who have elevated triglyceride levels [44]. Type 2 diabetes generally is associated with dyslipidemia that is composed of low HDL, high LDL, and hypertriglyceridemia. Fish oil supplementation in this pop-ulation has been proven statistically significant in lowering triglycerides by almost 30% without significantly increasing fasting glucose or hemoglobin A1c (HbA1c) [45]. The elderly population may benefit particularly from this intervention because, in addition to the obvious cardiovascular risks, elevated triglyceride levels are associated with poor cognitive performance evidenced by verbal fluency and impaired memory tasks [46].

A Mediterranean diet has been associated with decreased development of diabetes and other common chronic diseases. Although, as stated earlier, restrictive diets are not recommended in the geriatric population, the Mediterranean diet consists of high intake of unsaturated lipids, high intake of fiber, and a moderate intake of alcohol. In the European Prospective In-vestigation into Cancer and Nutrition-elderly study, a multicenter, prospec-tive cohort study investigating the role of several factors in cancer and other chronic disease, the findings in a cohort of participants aged 60 years or older support this theory. More than 70,000 men and women who did not have coronary artery disease, stroke, or cancer at enrollment completed information about their dietary intake. Adherence to Mediterranean diet was associated with lower overall mortality [47].

The evidence from past studies associating moderate or high alcohol intake with type 2 diabetes is conflicting, largely because of limited available data. A recent population-based study of elderly men using self-reported questionnaires in conjunction with euglycemic clamp techniques found no relation between self-estimated alcohol intake and insulin sensitivity but, as expected, did find an association between waist circumference and insulin sensitivity [48].

In the general population exercise training of moderate to high intensity has been proven to improve a patient's cardiac risk profile through improvement in body composition. The basis physiology involved is the shift from the use of a fatty acid source for muscle fuel to an energy source that includes muscle glycogen, circulating glucose, and fatty acids. This glucose use persists after the activity is ceased. Exercise is effective in reducing HbA1c independent of body mass [49]. Because of individual functional limitations, aerobic exercise may be difficult for the older patient. Resistance exercise is recommended in this population. Resistance exercise training improves body mass composition and increases conditioning and overall functional status. Increasing evidence shows the beneficial effects of resistance training, including glycemic and lipid control, in the geriatric patient [50–53].

Medical therapeutics of hyperglycemia

Therapeutics to decrease insulin resistance and prevent potential future complications of hyperglycemia in the long-term care population also can include alternate interventions, such as metformin, sulfonylureas, thiazolidinediones (TZDs), α-glucosidase inhibitors, and, more recently, modulators of the incretin system. Any drug benefit should be balanced and justified against the risk profile, which can be more enigmatic in the older population. To maintain patient safety and optimize patient care, ongoing research in drug therapies continues to be important, as seen presently with TZDs, as well as in newer drugs, such as exenatide and dipeptidyl peptidase IV (DPP IV) inhibitors.

Biguanides

Metformin is the sole available member of the biguanide class. It works to decrease hepatic glucose production while increasing hepatic glucose uptake, without having any effect on insulin secretion. Metformin is used widely in the general obese type 2 diabetic population for these hepatic effects. Anorexia and weight loss are also seen commonly, probably through inhibition of nitric oxide synthase [54–56]. Although weight loss is desirable in the obese younger patient, it is not desirable in the geriatric patient and leads to frailty. Metformin is not recommended for use in persons over the age of 80 years or in persons who have renal failure. Older persons frequently have muscle breakdown or sarcopenia that can mask renal insufficiency, further limiting its use in this population.

Sulfonylureas

The sulfonylureas are a class of drugs that target hyperglycemia by enhancing insulin secretion from the β cells of the pancreas. Their principle target is the ATP-sensitive potassium channel of the β-cell membrane. Inhibition of this channel by either glucose or sulfonylureas results in the triggering and opening of voltage-gated calcium channels, leading to calcium influx into the cell and insulin exocytosis. The members of this class are similar, varying mainly in half-life and potency based largely on the level of activity of the ATP potassium channel and its subunits. Sulfonylureas should be used cautiously in elderly patients and in any patient who has hepatic and renal failure, for fear of hypoglycemia.

Meglitinides

The meglitinides are a class of insulin secretagogues with rapid onset and short half-life are that often are used before meals to restore early-phase insulin release postprandially [57]. Available members are rapaglinide and nateglinide. In the general population these drugs often are used concurrently with metformin. The side effects of the meglitinides are similar to those of the sulfonylureas. These drugs should be used cautiously, if at all, in the geriatric patient.

Thiazolinediones

TZDs are a class of drugs that are both important and controversial in the treatment and understanding of diabetes today. They work via the PPAR-γ to promote insulin sensitivity at the level of the liver and muscle. The study of adipocytes and adipokines, especially adiponectin, has aided in the current understanding of insulin resistance and TZD pharmacology within recent years [58]. In the long-term care setting, insulin resistance is associated with a proinflammatory state [59]. An inverse association exists between adiponectin and insulin resistance, in that adiponectin enhances insulin-mediated repression of glucose production in the liver. In fact, adiponectin seems to enhance significantly the effects of even small amounts of insulin, as seen with the use of primary hepatocytes exposed in vitro to differing levels of insulin in the presence of absence of adiponectin [60]. Other than weight loss, the only current approach shown to increase adiponectin levels significantly is the use of activators of PPAR-γ [27]. These effects on insulin resistance have significant implications for the prevention of type 2 diabetes. The Diabetes Reduction Assessment With Ramipril and Rosiglitazone Medication trial showed that TZD treatment for 3 years resulted in substantial reductions in the incidence of diabetes in high-risk individuals [28]. Further studies have suggested some positive effects on atherosclerosis. Through ubiquitin-proteasome activity analysis, TZD treatment has been associated with decreased inflammation and resulting plaque stabilization in symptomatic carotid plaques [61]. Improvement in homocysteinemia in diabetic patients also was observed with the addition of this pharmacologic agent [62]. A growing amount of research, however, indicates possible consequences of PPAR-γ agonism on bone mineral density and should prompt clinicians to consider possible risks of accelerated bone loss and future fractures [63]. In vitro, TZD treatment seems to promote bone marrow progenitor cells toward adipogenesis rather than osteoblastogenesis [64], whereas observational studies support the hypothesis that TZDs are associated with and may cause bone loss in older women [65]. Additionally, recent research has emerged in regards to the long-term cardiovascular safety of TZDs, and data currently are being re-evaluated [66,67]. It seems that T2Ds may increase the risk of heart failure and possibly myocardial infarction in some susceptible individuals. This effect seems to be more likely with rosiglitazone than with pioglitazone. At present TZDs should be avoided in any person who has heart disease.

α-Glucosidase inhibitors

α-Glucosidase inhibitors are a class of drugs that target postprandial hyperglycemia by decreasing carbohydrate absorption at the intestinal brush border. The net result in elderly patients is greater insulin sensitivity as opposed to increased insulin release [68,69]. Currently available members of this drug class are acarbose and migitol. Recent studies suggest that these drugs also may increase glucagon-like peptide 1 (GLP-1), an incretin hormone that is discussed in more detail later [70,71]. The mechanism of action is unclear at this time. These drugs have a good overall safety profile for older populations; the most common side effects are gastrointestinal, such as bloating and loose stools, which unfortunately limit use in some patients. Postprandial hypotension is a significant clinical condition that predisposes elderly patients to events such as syncope and falls. Also, the severity of postprandial hypotension tends to be augmented by a greater carbohydrate content. The addition of α-glucosidase inhibitors seems to attenuate postprandial hypotension and its resulting effects [72–74].

Incretin mimetics and dipeptidyl peptidase IV inhibitors

The study of incretin hormones is adding to the available armamentarium of diabetic therapeutics. The gut hormones GLP-1 and gastric inhibitory polypeptide are incretin hormones that are released postprandially and increase glucose-stimulated insulin secretion through β-cell glucose sensitization. In healthy volunteers GLP-1 dose-dependently inhibits gastric emptying [75] and produces a fall in glucose representative of decreased hepatic glucose production, resulting from increased insulin and decreased glucagon secretion, as well as decreased entry of dietary carbohydrate into the small intestine [76]. Insulin resistance itself has a relationship with gastric motility and emptying, although the details are not completely clear. When IR-HOMA was used an index of insulin resistance in 20 nondiabetic subjects, the induction of hyperglycemia created significant bradygastria as determined by electrogastrography [77]. Inhibition of gastric emptying may itself cause a limitation of food intake through signaling pathways, neural or endocrine, secondary to gastric distention. Inhibition of food intake in rats is observed through intracerebroventricular GLP-1 administration through activation of brain GLP-1 receptors [78]. Human studies show GLP-1 enhances satiety and reduces energy intake, lending toward a role in appetite control [79]. Rapid insulin pulses and the orderliness of insulin release, known as entropy, seem to be disrupted in normal aging, as well as in disease states characterized by altered glucose metabolism, such as impaired glucose intolerance, obesity, and type 2 diabetes. The irregularity of insulin secretion is increased further in elderly patients who have diabetes relative to age-matched nondiabetic controls, but prolonged infusion of GLP-1 has been shown to improve to improve pulsatile insulin secretion in obese elderly patients who have type 2 diabetes [80]. GLP-1 has a short half-life of less than 1 minute, because it is rapidly degraded by the enzyme DPP IV.

The first clinically available incretin mimetic is exenatide, which has a half-life of 2.4 hours with clinical effects lasting up to 8 hours [81]. Exenatide has up to a 30-fold longer half-life and substantially greater glucose-lowering potential than GLP-1 [82]. Statistically significant reductions in HbA1c and both fasting and postprandial glucose levels, as well as body weight, have been recognized in placebo-controlled studies that added exenatide to the regimens of patients not achieving adequate control with metformin, a sulfonylurea, or both [83–85]. A recent study using a long-acting formulation, exenatide LAR, showed similar results [86]. The most common side effect noted in most studies is nausea, which probably contributes to the weight loss. This drug should not be used in older populations until more studies are available. Although studies have included older individuals, there are not adequate data specifically in these patients, especially concerning changes in body weight. Despite the benefits of improved glucose management, weight loss in the geriatric population, as mentioned earlier, generally is not beneficial and can lead to worsening frailty.

An alternate approach to increasing circulating levels of GLP-1, and thereby increasing the effects of GLP-1 on improved glucose homeostasis, is inhibition of DPP IV activity. In fact, DPP IV also degrades gastric inhibitory polypeptide, so its inhibition increases both major incretin hormones. In initial human studies, DPP IV inhibition in patients who had mild diabetes (HbA1c of 7.4%) showed improvements in fasting, postprandial, and 24-hour blood glucose levels and in insulin levels after only 4 weeks of treatment [87]. Subsequent studies showed no alterations in gastric emptying or a delayed rate of entry of ingested glucose into the circulation, as seen with administration of GLP-1 [88]. Therefore, DPP IV inhibitors improve glycemic control through stimulation of insulin secretion and inhibition of glucagon release. Sitagliptin is a highly selective oral DPP IV inhibitor. About 80% inhibition of DPP IV activity and a resulting doubled level of active GLP-1 were associated with a reduction in glucose levels after a glucose tolerance test in sitagliptin-treated lean rodents [89]. Sitagliptin treatment up to 600 mg generally was well tolerated without side effects, such as increased hypoglycemia or gastrointestinal complaints, compared with placebo in healthy euglycemic men [90]. In patients who had type 2 diabetes with inadequate glycemic control treated with metformin monotherapy, sitagliptin resulted in HbA1c reductions and a side-effect profile similar to that seen with sulfonylurea [91]. Considering the favorable gastrointestinal profile and the resulting effects on weight, as well as lack of hypoglycemia, the use of a DPP IV inhibitor would seem a reasonable therapeutic option for geriatric patients, even though there are no specific studies in this patient population. These agents are particularly useful because they do not seem to produce hypoglycemia.

Insulin resistance and fracture

Bone mineral density is known to decrease with age, leading to osteoporosis and its associated morbidity and mortality. Type 1 diabetes leads to decreased bone mineral density and increased fracture. After adjustment for hip bone mineral density, however, an increased risk of nontraumatic fracture has been observed in patients who have type 2 diabetes [92]. Postmenopausal women who have diabetes or who progress to develop diabetes also have been found to have a higher risk for hip fracture than postmenopausal women who do not diabetes [93]. Diabetes is considered an independent risk factor for hip fracture in elderly women [94]. Interestingly, in a recent study of elderly diabetic female nursing home residents, higher blood glucose levels were associated with decreased parathyroid hormone levels and decreased bone turnover [95]. Data have not clearly identified patients who have impaired glucose tolerance as being at increased for fracture at present [96].

Insulin resistance and hypogonadism

Hypogonadism may contribute to the prevalence of the insulin resistance syndrome [97]. The decline in testosterone levels associated with increased age has been a subject of recent research [98]. Furthermore, low testosterone levels have been associated with insulin resistance, which may improve upon testosterone replacement [99]. Although the initial association of low testosterone levels and diabetes risk often was confused by issues related to sex hormone-binding globulin, research has established an inverse relationship between insulin resistance and testosterone level independent of sex hormone-binding globulin [100]. This hypothesis is supported by studies of patients who had prostate cancer who, after treatment with gonadotropin-releasing hormone antagonist, developed glucose dysregulation and diabetes [101]. A recent cross-sectional study of diabetic men found, that on the basis of symptoms and biochemical evaluation, testosterone levels quite frequently were low in the setting of diabetes [102]. Given the potential concerns of metabolic syndrome, it is important to remember that low serum testosterone levels are associated with an increased risk of cardiovascular disease in men [103,104].

Summary

The incidence insulin resistance in the geriatric population is growing as this population grows. The management of hyperglycemia and its associated risk factors depends on an expanding understanding of the underlying pathophysiology and progression of disease and of currently available and future therapeutics, which are continually evolving. There is a major need for studies in the long-term care setting to determine the appropriate standard of care in prevention and treatment of metabolic dysregulation.

References

[1] Morley JE. Diabetes mellitus: a major disease of older persons. J Gerontol A Biol Sci Med Sci 2000;55:M255–6.

[2] Zarowitz BJ, Tangalos EG, Hollenack K, et al. The application of evidence-based principles of care in older persons (issue 3): management of diabetes mellitus. J Am Med Dir Assoc 2006;7:234–40.

[3] American Diabetes Association. Standards of medical care in diabetes. Diabetes Care 2006; 29:59–42.

[4] American Diabetes Association. Economic consequences of diabetes mellitus in the US in 2002. Diabetes Care 2003;26:917–32.

[5] Reaven GM. Role of insulin resistance in human disease. Diabetes 1988;37:1595–607.

[6] Johnson CL, Rifkind BM, Sempos CT, et al. Declining serum total cholesterol levels among US adults: the National Health and Nutrition Examination Surveys. JAMA 1993;269: 3002–8.

[7] Harris MI, Flegal KM, Cowie CC, et al. Prevalence of diabetes, impaired fasting glucose, and impaired glucose tolerance in US adults: the Third National Health and Nutrition Examination Survey, 1988–1994. Diabetes Care 1998;21:518–24.

[8] UK Prospective Diabetes Study Group. Intensive blood-glucose control with sulphonylureas or insulin compared with conventional treatment and risk of complications in patients with type 2 diabetes (UKPDS 33). Lancet 1998;352:837–53.

[9] Saydah S. Poor control of risk factors for vascular disease among adults with previously diagnosed diabetes mellitus. JAMA 2004;291:335–42.

[10] Executive summary of the third report of The National Cholesterol Education Program (NCEP) Expert Panel on Detection, Evaluation, and Treatment of High Blood Cholesterol in Adults (Adult Treatment Panel III). JAMA 2001;285:2486–97.

[11] Alberti KG, Zimmer PZ. Definition, diagnosis and classification of diabetes mellitus provisional report of a WHO consultation. Diabet Med 1998;15:539–53.

[12] Kahn R, Buse J, Ferrannini E, et al. The metabolic syndrome: time for a critical appraisal. Diabetes Care 2005;28:2289–304.

[13] Jeppesen J, Hansen TW, Rasmussen S, et al. Insulin resistance, the metabolic syndrome, and risk of incident cardiovascular disease: a population-based study. J Am Coll Cardiol 2007;49:2112–9.

[14] Nilsson G, Hedberg P, Jonason T, et al. Heart rate recovery is more strongly associated with the metabolic syndrome, waist circumference, and insulin sensitivity in women than in men among the elderly in the general population. Am Heart J 2007;154: 460.e1–7.

[15] Barzilay JI, Blaum C, Moore T, et al. Insulin resistance and inflammation as precursors of frailty: the Cardiovascular Health Study. Arch Intern Med 2007;167:635–41.

[16] Vogelzangs N, Beekman AT, Kritchevsky SB, et al. Psychosocial risk factors and the metabolic syndrome in elderly persons: finding from the health, aging and body composition study. J Gerontol A Biol Sci Med Sci 2007;62:563–9.

[17] Jackson RA. Mechanisms of age-related glucose intolerance. Diabetes Care 1990; 13(Suppl 2):9–19.

[18] De Rekeneire N, Peila R, Ding J, et al. Diabetes, hyperglycemia, and inflammation in older individuals. Diabetes Care 2006;29:1902–7.

[19] Beck-Nielsen H, Groop LC. Metabolic and genetic characterization of prediabetic states. Sequence of events leading to non-insulin-dependent diabetes mellitus. J Clin Invest 1994;94:1714–21.

[20] Stumvoll M, Goldstein BJ, van Haeften TW. Type 2 diabetes: principles of pathogenesis and therapy. Lancet 2005;365:1333–46.

[21] Petersen KF, Befroy D, Dufour S, et al. Mitochondrial dysfunction in the elderly: possible role in insulin resistance. Science 2003;300:1140–2.

[22] Figaro MK, Kritchevsky SB, Resnick HE, et al. Diabetes, inflammation, and function decline in older adults. Diabetes Care 2006;29:2039–45.

[23] Banks WE, Altmann J, Sapolsky RM, et al. Serum leptin levels as a marker for a syndrome X-like condition in wild baboons. J Clin Endocrinol Metab 2003;88:1234–40.

[24] Jacob S, Machann J, Rett K, et al. Association of increased intramyocellular lipid content with insulin resistance in lean nondiabetic offspring on type 2 diabetic subjects. Diabetes 1999;48:1113–9.

[25] Stefan N, Machann J, Schick F, et al. New imaging techniques of fat, muscle and liver within the context of determining insulin sensitivity. Horm Res 2005;64(Suppl 3): 38–44.

[26] Kershaw EE, Flier JS. Adipose tissue as an endocrine organ. J Clin Endocrinol Metab 2004; 89:2548–56.

[27] Berg AH, Combs TP, Du X, et al. The adipocyte-secreted protein Acrp30 enhances hepatic insulin action. Nat Med 2001;7:947–53.

[28] Combs TP, Wagner JA, Berger J, et al. Induction of adipocyte complement-related protein of 30 kilodaltons by PPARγ agonists: a potential mechanism of insulin sensitization. Endocrinology 2002;143:998–1007.

[29] Orchard TJ, Temprosa M, Goldberg R, et al. The effect of metformin and intensive lifestyle intervention on the metabolic syndrome: the Diabetes Prevention Program randomized trial. Ann Intern Med 2005;142:611–9.

[30] Diabetes Prevention Program Research Groups. Reduction in the incidence of type 2 diabetes with lifestyle intervention or metformin. N Engl J Med 2002;346:393–403.

[31] Tuomilehto J, Lindström J, Eriksson JG, et al. Prevention of type 2 diabetes mellitus by changes in lifestyle among subjects with impaired glucose tolerance. N Engl J Med 2001; 344:1343–50.

[32] Pan XR, Li GW, Hu YH, et al. Effects of diet and exercise in preventing NIDDM in people with impaired glucose tolerance: the Da Qing IGT and Diabetes Study. Diabetes Care 1997; 20:537–44.

[33] American Diabetes Association. Evidence-based nutrition principles and recommendation for the treatment and prevention of diabetes and related complication. Diabetes Care 2002; 25:202–12.

[34] American Diabetes Association. Nutrition recommendations and interventions for diabetes—2006. Diabetes Care 2006;29:2140–57.

[35] Morley JE, Kim MJ, Haren MT, et al. Frailty and the aging male. Aging Male 2005;8: 135–40.

[36] MacIntosh C, Morley JE, Chapman IM. The anorexia of aging. Nutrition 2000;16:983–95.

[37] Morley JE. Weight loss in the nursing home. J Am Med Dir Assoc 2007;8:201–4.

[38] Ensrud KE, Ewing SK, Taylor BC, et al. Frailty and risk of falls, fracture, and mortality in older women: the study of osteoporotic fractures. J Gerontol A Biol Sci Med Sci 2007;7: 744–51.

[39] Tariq SH, Karcic E, Thomas DR, et al. The use of no-concentrated-sweets diet in the management of type 2 diabetes in nursing homes. J Am Diet Assoc 2001;101:1463–6.

[40] Coulston AM, Mandelbaum D, Reaven GM. Dietary management of nursing home residents with non-insulin-dependent diabetes mellitus. Am J Clin Nutr 1990;51:67–71.

[41] Wedick NM, Barrett-Connor E, Knoke JD, et al. The relationship between weight loss and all-cause mortality in older men and women with and without diabetes mellitus: the Rancho Bernardo Study. J Am Geriatr Soc 2002;50:1810–5.

[42] American Diabetes Association. Nutrition recommendations and interventions for diabetes: a position statement of the American Diabetes Association. Diabetes Care 2007; 30(Suppl 1):S48–65.

[43] DeFillipis AP, Sperling LS. Understanding omega-3's. Am Heart J 2006;151:564–70.

[44] Marchioli R, Barzi F, Bomba E, et al. Early protection against sudden death by n-3 polyunsaturated fatty acids after myocardial infarction: time-course analysis of the results of the Gruppo Italiano per lo Studio della Sopravvivenza nell'Infarto Miocardico (GISSI)-Prevenzione. Circulation 2002;105:1897–903.

[45] Albert CM, Campos H, Stamper MJ, et al. Blood levels of long-chain n-3 fatty acids and the risk of sudden death. N Engl J Med 2002;346:1113–8.

[46] Rivellese A, Maffettone A, Iovine C, et al. Long-term effects of fish oil on insulin resistance and plasma lipoproteins in NIDDM patients with hypertriglyceridemia. Diabetes Care 1996;19:1207–11.

[47] Montori VM, Farmer A, Wollan PC, et al. Fish oil supplementation in type 2 diabetes. Diabetes Care 2000;23:1407–15.

[48] Friedberg C, Janssen MJ, Heine RJ, et al. Fish oil and glycemic control in diabetes. Diabetes Care 1998;21:494–500.

[49] Trichopoulou A, Orfanos P, Norat T, EPIC-Elderly Prospective Study Group. Modified Mediterranean diet and survival: EPIC-elderly prospective cohort study. BMJ 2005;330: 991–5.

[50] Riserus U, Ingelsson E. Alcohol intake, insulin resistance, and abdominal obesity in elderly men. Obesity 2007;15:1766–73.

[51] Sigal RJ, Kenny GP, Wasserman DH, et al. Physical activity/exercise and type 2 diabetes. Diabetes Care 2004;27:2518–37.

[52] Castaneda C, Layne JE, Munoz-Orians L, et al. A randomized controlled trial of resistance exercise training to improve glycemic control in older adults with type 2 diabetes. Diabetes Care 2002;25:2335–41.

[53] Dunstan DW, Daly RM, Owen N, et al. High-intensity resistance training improves glycemic control in older patients with type 2 diabetes. Diabetes Care 2002;25:1729–36.

[54] Kodama S, Shu M, Murakami H, et al. Even low-intensity and low-volume exercise training may improve insulin resistance in the elderly. Intern Med 2007;46:1071–7.

[55] Lee A, Morley JE. Metformin decreases food consumption and induces weight loss in subjects with obesity with type II non-insulin-dependent diabetes. Obes Res 1998;6: 47–53.

[56] Morley JE, Flood JF. Effect of competitive antagonism of NO synthetase on weight and food intake in obese and diabetic mice. Am J Physiol 1994;266(1 Pt 2):R164–8.

[57] Kumar VB, Bernardo AE, Vyas K, et al. Effect of metformin on nitric oxide synthase in genetically obese (ob/ob) mice. Life Sci 2001;69:2789–99.

[58] Dornshorst A. Insulinotropic meglitnide analogues. Lancet 2001;358:1709–16.

[59] Mazza AD, Morley JE. Metabolic syndrome in the older male population. Aging Male 2007;10:3–8.

[60] Banks WA, Willoughby LM, Thomas DR, et al. Insulin resistance syndrome in the elderly: assessment of functional, biochemical, metabolic, and inflammatory status. Diabetes Care 2007;29:2369–73.

[61] Gerstein HC, Yusuf S, Bosch J, et al. Effect of rosiglisb:last-page > tazone on the frequency of diabetes in patients with impaired glucose tolerance or impaired fasting glucose: a randomized controlled trial. Lancet 2006;368:1096–105.

[62] Marfella R, D'Amico M, Di Filippo C, et al. Increased activity of the ubiquitin-proteasome system in patients with symptomatic carotid disease is associated with enhanced inflammation and may destabilize the atherosclerotic plaque: effects of rosiglitazone treatment. J Am Coll Cardiol 2006;47:2444–55.

[63] Cicero DG, D'Angelo A, Gaddi A, et al. Effects of 1 year of treatment with pioglitazone or rosiglitazone added to glimepiride on lipoprotein (a) and homocysteine concentrations in patients with type 2 diabetes mellitus and metabolic syndrome: a multicenter, randomized, double-blind, controlled clinical trial. Clin Ther 2006;28:679–88.

[64] Grey A. Skeletal consequences of thiazolidinedione therapy. Osteoporos Int 2007;19: 129–37.

[65] Crosson JT, Majika SM, Grazia T, et al. Rosiglitazone promotes development of a novel adipocyte population from bone marrow-derived circulating progenitor cells. J Clin Invest 2006;116:3220–8.

[66] Schwartz AV, Sellmeyer DE, Vittinghoff E, et al. Thiazolidinedione use and bone loss in older diabetic adults. J Clin Endocrinol Metab 2006;91:3349–54.

[67] Nissen NE, Wolski K. Effect of rosiglitazone on the risk of myocardial infarction and death from cardiovascular causes. N Engl J Med 2007;356:2457–71.

[68] Home PD, Pocock ST, Beck-Nielsen H, et al. Rosiglitazone evaluated for cardiovascular outcomes—an interim analysis. N Engl J Med 2007;357:28–38.

[69] Meneilly GS, Ryan EA, Radziuk J, et al. Effect of acarbose on insulin sensitivity in elderly patients with diabetes. Diabetes Care 2000;23:1162–7.

[70] Josse RG, Chiasson JL, Ryan EA, et al. Acarbose in the treatment of elderly patients with type 2 diabetes. Diabetes Res Clin Pract 2003;59:37–42.

[71] Lee A, Patrick P, Wishart J, et al. The effects of miglitol on glucagon-like peptide-1 secretion and appetite sensations in obese type 2 diabetics. Diabetes Obes Metab 2002;4: 329–35.

[72] DeLeon MJ, Chandurkar V, Albert SG, et al. Glucagon-like peptide-1 response to acarbose in elderly type 2 diabetic subjects. Diabetes Res Clin Pract 2002;56:101–6.

[73] Gentilcore D, Bryant B, Wishart JM, et al. Acarbose attenuates the hypotensive response to sucrose and slows gastric emptying in the elderly. Am J Med 2005;118:1289.

[74] Morley JE. Editorial: postprandial hypotension—the ultimate Big Mac attack. J Gerontol A Biol Sci Med Sci 2001;56:M741–3.

[75] Shibao C, Gamboa A, Diedrich A, et al. Acarbose, an α-glucosidase inhibitor, attenuates postprandial hypotension in autonomic failure. Hypertension 2007;50:54–61.

[76] Nauck MA, Niedereichholz U, Ettler R, et al. Glucagon-like peptide 1 inhibition of gastric emptying outweighs its insulinotropic effects in healthy humans. Am J Physiol 1997;273: 981–8.

[77] Hvidberg A, Nielsen MT, Hilsted J, et al. Effect of glucagon-like peptide 1 (proglucagon 78-107 amide) on hepatic glucose production in healthy men. Metabolism 1994;43:104–8.

[78] Kaji M, Nomura M, Tamura Y, et al. Relationships between insulin resistance, blood glucose levels and gastric motility: an electrogastrography and external ultrasonography study. J Med Invest 2007;54:168–76.

[79] Tang-Christensen M, Larsen PJ, Goke R, et al. Central administration of GLP-1-(7-36) amide inhibits food and water intake in rats. Am J Physiol 1996;271:848–56.

[80] Flint A, Raben A, Astrup A, et al. Glucagon-like peptide 1 promotes satiety and suppresses energy intake in humans. J Clin Invest 1998;101:515–20.

[81] Meneilly GS, Veldhuis JD, Elahi D. Deconvolution analysis of rapid insulin pulses before and after six weeks of continuous subcutaneous administration of glucagon-like peptide-1 in elderly patients with type 2 diabetes. J Clin Endocrinol Metab 2004;90:6251–6.

[82] Egan JM, Clocquet AR, Elahi D. The insulinotropic effect of acute exendin-4 administered to humans: comparison of nondiabetic state to type 2 diabetes. J Clin Endocrinol Metab 2002;87:1282–90.

[83] Nielsen LL, Young AA, Parkes DG. Pharmacology of exenatide (synthetic exendin-4): a potential therapeutic for improved glycemic control of type 2 diabetes. Regul Pept 2004;117:77–88.

[84] DeFronzo RA, Ratner RE, Han J, et al. Effects of exenatide (exendin-4) on glycemic control and weight over 30 weeks in metformin-treated patients with type 2 diabetes. Diabetes Care 2005;28:1092–100.

[85] Buse JB, Henry RR, Han J, et al. Exenatide-113 Clinical Study Group. Effects of exenatide (exendin-4) on glycemic control over 30 weeks in sulfonylurea-treated patients with type 2 diabetes. Diabetes Care 2004;27:2628–35.

[86] Kendall DM, Riddle MC, Rosenstock J, et al. Effects of exenatide (exendin-4) on glycemic control over 30 weeks in patients with type 2 diabetes treated with metformin and a sulfonylurea. Diabetes Care 2005;28:1083–91.

[87] Kim D, MacDonell L, Zhuang D, et al. Effects of once-weekly dosing of a long-acting release formulation of exenatide on glucose control and body weight in subjects with type 2 diabetes. Diabetes Care 2006;30:1487–93.

[88] Ahren B, Simonsson E, Larsson H, et al. Inhibition of dipeptidyl peptidase IV improves metabolic control over a 4-week study period in type 2 diabetes. Diabetes Care 2002;25: 869–75.

[89] Vella A, Bock G, Giesler PD, et al. Effects of dipeptidyl peptidase-4 inhibition on gastrointestinal function, meal appearance, and glucose metabolism in type 2 diabetes. Diabetes 2007;56:1475–80.

[90] Kim D, Wang L, Beconi M, et al. (2R)-4-oxo-4-[3-(trifluoromethyl)-5,6-dihydro[1,2,4]triazolo[4,3-a]pyrazin-7(8H)-yl]1-(2,4,5-trifluorophenyl)butan-2-amine: a potent, orally active dipeptidyl peptidase IV inhibitor for the treatment of type 2 diabetes. J Med Chem 2005;48: 141–51.

[91] Herman GA, Stevens C, Van Dyck K, et al. Pharmacokinetics and pharmacodynamics of single doses of sitagliptin, an inhibitor of dipeptidyl peptidase-IV, in healthy subjects. Clin Pharmacol Ther 2005;78:675–88.

[92] Nauck MA, Meininger G, Sheng D, et al. Efficacy and safety of the dipeptidyl peptidase-4 inhibitor, sitagliptin, compared with the sulfonylurea, glipizide, in patients with type 2 diabetes inadequately controlled on metformin alone: a randomized, double-blind, noninferiority trial. Diabetes Obes Metab 2007;9:194–205.

[93] Strotmeyer ES, Cauley JA, Schwartz AV, et al. Nontraumatic fracture risk with diabetes mellitus and impaired fasting glucose in older white and black adults: the health, aging, and body composition study. Arch Intern Med 2005;165:1612–7.

[94] Nicodemus KK, Folsom AR. Type 1 and type 2 diabetes and incident hip fractures in postmenopausal women. Diabetes Care 2001;24:1192–7.

[95] Taylor BC, Schreiner PJ, Stone KL, et al. Long-term prediction of incident hip fracture risk in elderly white women: study of osteoporotic fractures. J Am Geriatr Soc 2004;52:1479–86.

[96] Dobnig H, Piswanger-Solkner JC, Roth M, et al. Type 2 diabetes mellitus in nursing home patients: effects on bone turnover, bone mass, and fracture risk. J Clin Endocrinol Metab 2006;91:3355–63.

[97] de Liefde II, van der Klift M, de Laet CE, et al. Bone mineral density and fracture risk in type-2 diabetes mellitus: the Rotterdam Study. Osteoporos Int 2005;16:1713–20.

[98] Rodriguez A, Muller DC, Metter EJ, et al. Aging, androgens, and the metabolic syndrome in a longitudinal study of aging. J Clin Endocrinol Metab 2007;92:3568–78.

[99] Travison TG, Morley JE, Araujo AB, et al. The relationship between libido and testosterone levels in aging men. J Clin Endocrinol Metab 2005;91:2509–13.

[100] Kapoor D, Aldred H, clark S, et al. Clinical and biochemical assessment of hypogonadism in men with type 2 diabetes. Diabetes Care 2007;30:911–7.

[101] Tsai EC, Matsumoto AM, Fujimoto WY, et al. Association of bioavailable, free, and total testosterone with insulin resistance. Diabetes Care 2004;27:861–8.

[102] Basaria S, Muller DC, Carducci MA, et al. Hyperglycemia and insulin resistance in men with prostate carcinoma who receive androgen-deprivation therapy. Cancer 2006;106:581–8.

[103] Fukui M, Kitagawa Y, Nakamura N, et al. Association between serum testosterone concentration in men with type 2 diabetes. Diabetes Care 2003;26:1869–73.

[104] Kapoor D, Goodwin E, Channer KS, et al. Testosterone replacement therapy improves insulin resistance, glycaemic control, visceral adiposity and hypercholesterolaemia in hypogonadal men with type 2 diabetes. Eur J Endocrinol 2006;154:899–906.

ELSEVIER
SAUNDERS

CLINICS IN
GERIATRIC
MEDICINE

Clin Geriatr Med 24 (2008) 455–469

Diabetes, Sarcopenia, and Frailty

John E. Morley, MB, BCh[a,b,*]

[a]*Geriatric Research Education and Clinical Center, St. Louis VA Medical Center, 1 Jefferson Barracks Drive, 11E, St. Louis, MO 63125, USA*
[b]*Geriatric Medicine, Saint Louis University School of Medicine, 1402 S. Grand Boulevard, Room M238, St. Louis, MO 63104-1079, USA*

Persons who have diabetes mellitus tend to have an accelerated aging process [1,2] that places them at greater risk for developing frailty at an earlier age [3–10]. Frailty can be defined simply as a condition in which an older person is coping just above the disability threshold, but any stressor (either physical or psychologic) is liable to cause the person to become disabled or need intensive long-term physical therapy to allow recovery to the pre-disability state [6]. Rockwood and colleagues [11–13] have stressed that frailty really is the sum total of the number of illnesses a person has resulting in a physical decline. An objective definition of frailty created by Fried and her colleagues [14] has been validated and includes five components:

- Unintentional weight loss (10 pounds within the last year)
- Self-reported exhaustion
- Weakness (grip strength)
- Slow walking speed
- Low physical activity

The International Academy of Nutrition Health and Aging has operationalized the definition of frailty combining components of both Rockwood's and Fried's definitions [15,16] in the acronym "FRAIL":

Fatigue
Resistance (cannot climb one flight of stairs)
Ambulation (cannot walk one block)
Illnesses (more than five)
Loss of weight (< 5% over 1 year or less)

---

* Geriatric Medicine, Saint Louis University School of Medicine, 1402 S. Grand Blvd., Room M238, St. Louis, MO 63104-1079.
E-mail address: morley@slu.edu

0749-0690/08/$ - see front matter. Published by Elsevier Inc.
doi:10.1016/j.cger.2008.03.004

Overall, the presence of frailty depends on deterioration in muscle and nerve function, anemia, declining cardiopulmonary reserve, and loss of executive function [15,16]. Diabetes mellitus tends to cause problems in each of these areas. Insulin resistance is a key factor in the failure of many of these systems [17] and has been shown to relate to excess disability in nursing home residents [18]. Loss of homeostasis occurs commonly in diabetic persons and leads to vulnerability, a construct similar to that of frailty. In the end, frailty results in increased institutionalization, hospitalization, and mortality.

Falls, fractures, and frailty

Falls are a common problem in frail older persons. In the study of osteoporotic fractures of 9249 women, 18% of women fell more than once a year [19]. Non-insulin–treated diabetics had an age-associated increased risk of falls (odds ratio, 2.78), as did insulin-treated diabetics (odds ratio, 1.668). Diabetics who fell had more falls than nondiabetics. In the non-insulin–dependent diabetic women, the increased falls could be explained by an increase in factors known to increase the risk for falls. This was not the case for falls in insulin-dependent diabetics. Tilling and colleagues [20] found that the incidence of falls in older persons who had diabetes was 39%. Risk factors for falls in this group were poor diabetic control, needing assistance with mobility, and a prior cerebrovascular accident. In the Women's Health and Aging Study, women who had diabetes also had a higher propensity for falling and for having more than one fall compared with women who did not have diabetes [21]. Risk factors for falls included musculoskeletal pain, insulin therapy, obesity, and poor lower extremity performance. Miller and colleagues [22] found that older diabetic persons were at increased risk for both falls and injurious falls.

In a nursing home study, 35% of residents fell during a period of 299 days. The incidence of falling was 78% for diabetics and 30% for nondiabetics. Only abnormal gait and balance and diabetes independently predicted falls [23].

Patients who have type 1 diabetes have poor bone formation related to the decreased anabolic effects of insulin [24]. Therefore these patients are more likely to be osteopenic. Patients who have type 2 diabetic tend to have higher bone mineral density, although thiazolidinediones have been shown to produce osteopenia [25]. Despite greater bone mineral density, women who have type 2 diabetes mellitus have an increased risk of fracture.

Bonds and colleagues [26] studied 93,676 postmenopausal women in the Women's Health Initiative Observational Cohort. They found that women who had diabetes had an increased odds ratio of fractures of 1.20 after correcting for fall frequency. In nearly 3000 women between the ages of 70 and 79 years, diabetes mellitus carried an elevated risk of fracture of 1.64 after correcting for risk factors for fracture [27]. Those who experienced fracture had lower bone mineral density and lean mass, reduced peripheral sensation, an increased incidence of stroke, and more falls.

A major risk factor for hip fracture in older persons is vitamin D deficiency [28–30], which is associated with osteopenia and also with increased falls [31,32]. Recent studies have clearly shown the vitamin D needs to be replaced aggressively when 25-hydroxy (25[OH]D) vitamin D levels are less than 30 ng/mL [33–37]. Vitamin 25(OH)D levels decline longitudinally with aging [38]. Vitamin D levels are lower in diabetics than in nondiabetics [39].

Testosterone levels in older males often are in the hypogonadal range [40–43]. Men who have diabetes have lower testosterone and bioavailable testosterone levels than do nondiabetic men [44,45]. Low testosterone levels are associated with increased falls and hip fractures [46,47]. Testosterone replacement therapy increased muscle mass and strength, bone mineral density, and function [48–51].

Two important causes of falls in older diabetics that often are overlooked are orthostasis and postprandial hypotension [52–54]. All older diabetics should have their blood pressure measured while standing. Aggressive treatment of orthostasis is important, and these patients may need treatment with midodrine or fludrocortisone. Postprandial hypotension occurs when a meal releases vasodilatory peptides such as calcitonin gene–related peptide, resulting in falls, syncope, and/or myocardial infarction [55]. The alpha-1-glucosidase inhibitors release glucagon-like peptide 1 which slows gastric emptying [56]. Slowing the rate of gastric emptying decreases the fall in blood pressure following a meal [57]. Both miglitol and acarbose can be used to decrease postprandial hypotension [58].

Osteoporosis is poorly recognized and treated by physicians [59,60]. In diabetics there is a need to look actively for osteoporosis and provide aggressive treatment with calcium, vitamin D, and bisphosphonates [61–64]. Elderly women who have diabetes mellitus may be resistant to bisphosphonates [65].

Sarcopenia

Diabetic patients tend to have worse function than nondiabetics [22,66–68]. This impairment is associated with a decline in muscle function. Persons who have diabetes mellitus, particularly when associated with renal failure, have accelerated loss of muscle function [68–71]. Different factors predict loss of muscle mass and decline in muscle strength [72].

Sarcopenia is the age-related decline in muscle mass [73]. It has been defined operationally as appendicular lean mass divided by height squared [74]. Sarcopenia is associated with increased disability and mortality [75]. Fat infiltration into muscle can be demonstrated by attenuation on muscle MRI [76]. This fat infiltration is termed "myosteatosis" and may play a major role in the decline in muscle strength with aging. Persons who have excess fat and sarcopenic muscles—the sarcopenic obese or "fat frail" patients—have very high levels of disability and mortality [77].

The causes of sarcopenia are multifactorial (Table 1) [78]. Free fatty acid accumulation within tissue leads to abnormalities in phosphorylation of the insulin receptor substrate and function of the glucose transporter receptor [79]. This accumulation can occur because of abnormalities in mitochondria or increased circulating triglycerides. Altered glucose metabolism leads to decreased muscle strength.

Diabetes is associated with peripheral neuropathy and a decrease in motor end plates [80]. Motor end plates play an important role in maintaining muscle mass and coordinating muscle contraction. Thus, their loss plays an important role in the pathogenesis of loss of muscle function.

Anabolic hormones are important in the maintenance of muscle mass by activating the phosphotidyl-inositol-3-kinase–active human protein kinase system in the cell [81]. Insulin resistance decreases the activity of this pathway. Growth hormone increases insulin growth factor-1 (IGF-1) that plays a major role in increased protein synthesis and decreased protein catabolism. A gene-splice variant of IGF-1 called "mechanogrowth factor" plays an important role in stimulating satellite cells and repair of motor units [82].

The decline in IGF-1 in diabetic animal models results in a sixfold increase in atrogene activation with a subsequent increase in proteolysis [83]. Increasing IGF-1 levels restored the atrogenes to normal levels.

Testosterone and dehydroepiandrosterone sulfate are both related to muscle mass and strength [84–87]. The low levels of bioavailable testosterone in diabetic and ageing men play an important role in the loss of muscle mass and strength [88–90]. Besides direct effects on protein synthesis, possibly by increasing IGF-1, testosterone also stimulates stem cells to produce satellite

Table 1
Factors involved in the pathogenesis of sarcopenia

Factor	Effect of aging	Effect of diabetes	Major systems altered
Motor end plates	Decrease	Decrease	Coordinated muscle contraction
Insulin growth factor-1	Decrease	Decrease	Protein synthesis
Mechanogrowth factor	Decrease	Unknown	Satellite cell formation
Ghrelin	Uncertain	Decrease	Anorexia and growth hormone
Testosterone	Decrease	Decrease	Protein synthesis and satellite formation
Myostatin	Unknown	None	Inhibits satellite cell formation and proteolysis
Proinflammatory cytokines	Increase	Increase	Proteolysis and apoptosis
Angiotensin	None	Increase	Cleaves actinomycin
Oxidative metabolism	Decrease	Increase	Oxidative damage
Food intake	Decrease	Increase	Muscle and fat
Creatine/branched chain amino acids	Decrease	Decrease	Protein synthesis
Exercise	Decrease	Mostly decrease	Protein synthesis

cells and inhibit the production of adipocytes [91]. Satellite availability is essential to allow muscle repair and to maintain muscle strength.

Ghrelin is a peptide hormone produced from the fundus of the stomach. It increases food intake, growth hormone release, and memory [92,93]. Ghrelin levels are lower in persons who have type 2 diabetes mellitus, suggesting a possible role for ghrelin in the regulation of muscle mass [94].

Myostatin is a protein that inhibits muscle growth [95]. It both inhibits satellite cell cycling and, through cachexia-inducing factor, increases proteolysis. Its levels are not altered in diabetes [96].

Proinflammatory cytokines such as tumor necrosis factor alpha and interleukin-6 play an important role in stimulating proteolysis and apoptosis in muscle cells [97]. Cytokines stimulate proteolysis by activating muscle ring finger protein-1, which then results in activation of the ubiquitin-proteasome system (the "intracellular death chamber"). This activation leads to the formation of amino acids and small peptides that are exported from the muscle into the circulation. There is a strong correlation between interleukin-6 and muscle mass, strength, and functional status [98,99]. Persons who have diabetes have elevated cytokine levels, suggesting that cytokines play an important role in the development of the sarcopenia associated with diabetes [100].

Diabetes results in elevated angiotensin II levels [101]. Angiotensin II activates capsases that cleave actin from myosin. This cleavage represents the first step in muscle breakdown. Cleavage of actin from myosin is essential before these proteins can undergo proteolysis by the ubiquitin-proteasome system. Angiotensin-converting enzyme inhibitors are associated with increased strength [102].

Diabetes have elevated levels of oxidative metabolism [103] that can lead to liposomal damage of the cells and apoptosis. In addition, declining levels of phosphocreatine reduce energy transfer from the mitochondria. Creatine replacement together with exercise increased muscle strength in older persons [104,105].

Weight loss caused by poor nutritional status leads to muscle wasting [106,107]. With aging there is a physiologic anorexia of aging that places older persons at risk of developing severe weight loss and muscle atrophy when they have a superimposed disease [108–113]. Maintenance of muscle mass requires relatively high protein intake on the order of 1.2 to 1.5 g/kg [114]. Because of fears of renal disease, diabetics often receive too little protein in their diet. Branched-chain amino acids such as leucine play an important role in the maintenance of protein synthesis because they stimulate mammalian target of rapamycin, which increases the rate of protein synthesis and decreases hysosomal activity.

Muscle hypoxia plays an important role in sarcopenia. Atherosclerosis decreases blood flow to the leg muscles resulting in decreased strength and exercise capacity [115,116]. Anemia occurs commonly in older persons, especially in those who have some degree of renal failure [31,106,117–119].

Immobility and decreased physical activity play a major role in the loss of muscle activity. Disuse activity occurs rapidly in older persons at bed rest [120]. Exercise, particularly resistance exercise, plays a key role in the maintenance of muscle mass [121–124].

Fig. 1 provides a simplified view of the biochemical changes in muscle in older diabetics that lead to the loss of muscle mass.

The treatment of sarcopenia in diabetics requires a multifocal approach, as outlined in Fig. 2.

Executive function

A decline in executive function predicts functional decline and mortality [125]. Executive function can decline acutely in persons who have delirium [126]. Diabetics can develop delirium related to hyper- or hypoglycemia

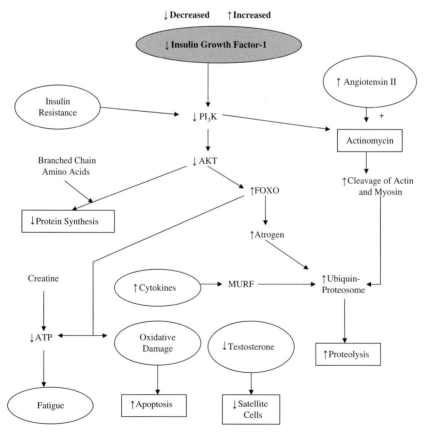

Fig. 1. Biochemical changes in muscle in diabetes. ↓, decreased; ↑, increased; KT, active human protein kinase (protein kinase-B); FOXO, forkhead protein; MURF, muscle ring finger protein; PI3K, phosphatidyl inositol-3-kinase.

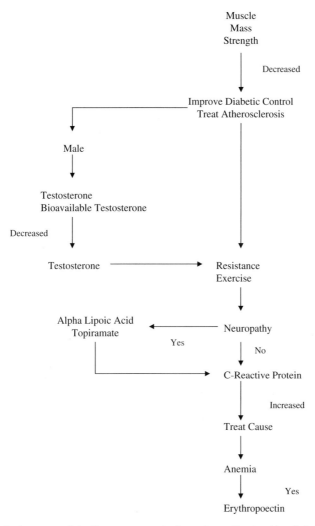

Fig. 2. An approach to the management of muscle wasting in older diabetics.

or hypertriglyceridemia [126,127] or from any of the other causes of delirium.

Numerous studies have shown that dementia occurs more commonly in diabetics than in persons who do not have diabetes [128–132]. Persons who have diabetes are at increased risk for developing vascular dementia. In addition, there is some evidence that diabetics are more likely to develop Alzheimer's disease [133,134]. The enzymes that degrade insulin also degrade amyloid beta protein [135]. It has been suggested that elevated insulin levels result in decreased degradation of amyloid beta protein. Amyloid beta protein has been shown to decrease cognition directly [136–138]. The direct effects of insulin on memory are controversial.

Saint Louis University
Mental Status (SLUMS) Examination

Name _____ Age _____
Is patient alert? _____ Level of education _____

__/1	❶	1. What day of the week is it?
__/1	❶	2. What is the year?
__/1	❶	3. What state are we in?

4. Please remember these five objects. I will ask you what they are later.
　　　Apple　　　Pen　　　Tie　　　House　　　Car

5. You have $100 and you go to the store and buy a dozen apples for $3 and a tricycle for $20.
❶　　How much did you spend?
__/3　❷　　How much do you have left?

6. Please name as many animals as you can in one minute.
__/3　　❶ 0-4 animals　❶5-9 animals　❷10-14 animals　❸15+ animals

__/5　7. What were the five objects I asked you to remember? 1 point for each one correct.

8. I am going to give you a series of numbers and I would like you to give them to me backwards.
For example, if I say 42, you would say 24.
__/2　　❶ 87　　❶ 649　　❶ 8537

9. This is a clock face. Please put in the hour markers and the time at
ten minutes to eleven o'clock.
❷　Hour markers okay
__/4　❷　Time correct
__/2　❶ 10. Please place an X in the triangle.

❶　Which of the above figures is largest?

11. I am going to tell you a story. Please listen carefully because afterwards, I'm going to ask you
some questions about it.
Jill was a very successful stockbroker. She made a lot of money on the stock market. She then met
Jack, a devastatingly handsome man. She married him and had three children. They lived in Chicago.
She then stopped work and stayed at home to bring up her children. When they were teenagers, she
went back to work. She and Jack lived happily ever after.
❷ What was the female's name?　　　　❷ What work did she do?
❷ When did she go back to work?　　　❷ What state did she live in?

__/8

_____　TOTAL SCORE

SAINT LOUIS
UNIVERSITY

SCORING		
HIGH SCHOOL EDUCATION		LESS THAN HIGH SCHOOL EDUCATION
27-30	Normal	20-30
20-26	MCI	15-19
1-19	Dementia	1-14

WA Banks and JE Morley. Memories are made of this: Recent advances in understanding, cognitive impairment, and dementia. *J Gerontol Med Sci* 2003;58A:314–21.

Fig. 3. Saint Louis University Mental Status examination. (*From* Banks WA, Morley JA. Memories are made of this: recent advances in understanding, cognitive impairment, and dementia. J Gerontol Med Sci 2003;58A:317; with permission.)

Diabetics are at increased risk of developing depression [139]. Depression interferes with executive function and can result in weight loss and increased hospitalization and death in older persons [140–142].

For these reasons it is important to screen older persons who have diabetes regularly for cognitive dysfunction. This screening can be done successfully with the Saint Louis University Mental Status examination (Fig. 3) [143,144]. This test successfully recognizes amnestic mild cognitive dysfunction as well as dementia.

The treatment of executive dysfunction in diabetes involves control of glycemia and hypertension and the use of aspirin to prevent future strokes. Drugs available to treat dementia (ie, the cholinesterase inhibitors and memantine) may help some persons, but their efficacy is limited [145–148]. Animal studies have suggested that free radical scavengers, such as alpha-lipoic acid, may improve cognition [149,150].

Summary

Frailty is a pre-disability condition. It now can be defined clinically. The major factors leading to frailty are sarcopenia and a decline in executive function. Stressors precipitate frail individuals into a state of disability. Diabetics develop the conditions necessary for frailty earlier than other aging individuals. Appropriate treatment of diabetes mellitus and frailty precursors can result in a slowing of the aging process.

References

[1] Kim MJ, Rolland Y, Cepeda O, et al. Diabetes mellitus in older men. Aging Male 2006;9: 139–47.
[2] Mazza AD, Morley JE. Update on diabetes in the elderly and the application of current therapeutics. J Am Med Dir Assoc 2007;8:489–92.
[3] Morley JE, Haren MT, Rolland Y, et al. Frailty. Med Clin North Am 2006;90:837–47.
[4] Fried LP, Ferrucci L, Darer J, et al. Untangling the concepts of disability, frailty, and comorbidity: implications for improved targeting and care. J Gerontol A Biol Sci Med Sci 2004;59:255–63.
[5] Morley JE, Kim MJ, Haren MT, et al. Frailty and the aging male. Aging Male 2005;8: 135–40.
[6] Morley JE, Perry HM, Miller DK. Something about frailty. J Gerontol A Biol Sci Med Sci 2002;57:M698–704.
[7] Whitson HE, Purser JL, Cohen HJ. Frailty thy name is...phrailty? J Gerontol A BIol Sci Med Sci 2007;62:728–30.
[8] Kahn AJ. Central and peripheral mechanisms of aging and frailty: a report on the 8th Longevity Consortium Symposium, Santa Fe, New Mexico, May 16–18, 2007. J Gerontol A BIol Sci Med Sci 2007;62:1357–60.
[9] Haas LB. Optimizing insulin use in type 2 diabetes: role of basal and prandial insulin in long-term care facilities. J Am Med Dir Assoc 2007;8:502–10.
[10] Zarowitz BJ, Tangalos EG, Hollenack K, et al. The application of evidence-based principles of care in older persons (issue 3): management of diabetes mellitus. J Am Med Dir Assoc 2006;7:234–40.
[11] Rockwood K. Frailty and its definition: a worthy challenge. J Am Geriatr Soc 2005;53: 1069–70.
[12] Rockwood K, Abeysundera MJ, Mitnitski A. How should we grade frailty in nursing home patients? J Am Med Dir Assoc 2007;8:595–603.
[13] Jones D, Song X, Mitnitski A, et al. Evaluation of a frailty index based on a comprehensive geriatric assessment in a population based study of elderly Canadians. Aging Clin Exp Res 2005;17:464–71.

[14] Fried LP, Tangen CM, Walston J, et al. Frailty in older adults: evidence for a phenotype. J Gerontol A Biol Sci Med Sci 2001;56:M146–56.

[15] Abellan van Kan A, Rolland Y, Bergman H, et al. Frailty assessment of older people in clinical practice: expert opinion of a geriatric advisory panel. J Nutr Health Aging 2008; 12:29–37.

[16] Abellan van Kan G, Rolland YM, Morley JE, et al. Frailty: toward a clinical definition. J Am Med Dir Assoc 2008;9:71–2

[17] Mazza AD, Morley JE. Metabolic syndrome and the older male population. Aging Male 2007;10:3–8.

[18] Banks WA, Willoughby LM, Thomas DR, et al. Insulin resistance syndrome in the elderly: assessment of functional, biochemical, metabolic, and inflammatory status. Diabetes Care 2007;30:2369–73.

[19] Schwartz AV, Hillier TA, Sellmeyer DE, et al. Older women with diabetes have a higher risk of falls: a prospective study. Diabetes Care 2002;25:1749–54.

[20] Tilling LM, Darawil K, Britton M. Falls as a complication of diabetes mellitus in older people. J Diabetes Complications 2006;20:158–62.

[21] Volpato S, Leveille SG, Blaum C, et al. Risk factors for falls in disabled women with diabetes: the women' health and aging study. J Gerontol A Biol Sci Med Sci 2005;60: 1539–45.

[22] Miller DK, Lui LY, Perry HM 3rd, et al. Reported and measured physical functioning in older inner-city diabetic African-Americans. J Gerontol A Biol Sci Med Sci 1999;54: M230–6.

[23] Maurer MS, Burcham J, Cheng H. Diabetes mellitus is associated with an increased risk of falls in elderly residents of a long-term care facility. J Gerontol A Biol Sci Med Sci 2005;60: 1157–62.

[24] Hofbauer LC, Brueck CC, Singh SK, et al. Osteoporosis in patients with diabetes mellitus. J Bone Miner Res 2007;22:1317–28.

[25] Schwartz AV, Sellmeyer DE. Diabetes, fracture, and bone fragility. Curr Osteoporos Rep 2007;5:105–11.

[26] Bonds DE, Larson JC, Schwartz AV, et al. Risk of fracture in women with type 2 diabetes: the Women's Health Initiative Observational Study. J Clin Endocrinol Metab 2006;91: 3404–10.

[27] Strotmeyer ES, Cauley JA, Schwartz AV, et al. Nontraumatic fracture risk with diabetes mellitus and impaired fasting glucose in older white and black adults: the health, aging, and body composition study. Arch Intern Med 2005;165:1612–7.

[28] Duque G, Mallet L, Roberts A, et al. To treat or not to treat, that is the question: proceedings of the Quebec symposium for the treatment of osteoporosis in long-term care institutions. Saint Hyacinthe, Quebec, November 5, 2004. J Am Med Dir Assoc 2007; 8(3 Suppl 2):e67–73.

[29] Zarowitz BJ, Stefanacci R, Hollenack K, et al. The application of evidence-based principles of care in older persons (issue 1): management of osteoporosis. J Am Med Dir Assoc 2007; 8(3 Suppl 2):e51–7.

[30] Messinger-Rapport BJ, Morley JE, Thomas DR, et al. Intensive session: new approaches to medical issues in long-term care. J Am Med Dir Assoc 2007;8:421–33.

[31] Dharmarajan TS. Falls and fractures linked to anemia, delirium, osteomalacia, medications and more: the path to success is strewn with obstacles!. J Am Med Dir Assoc 2007; 8:549–50.

[32] Morley JE. Should all long-term care residents receive vitamin D? J Am Med Dir Assoc 2007;8:69–70.

[33] Drinka PJ, Krause PF, Nest LJ, et al. Determinants of vitamin D levels in nursing home residents. J Am Med Dir Assoc 2007;8:76–9.

[34] Munir J, Wright RJ, Carr DB. A quality improvement study on calcium and vitamin D supplementation in long term care. J Am Med Dir Assoc 2007;8(3 Suppl 2):e19–23.

[35] Hamid Z, Riggs A, Spencer T, et al. Vitamin D deficiency in residents of academic long-term care facilities despite having been prescribed vitamin D. J Am Med Dir Assoc 2007; 8:71–5.

[36] Wright RM. Use of osteoporosis medications in older nursing facility residents. J Am Med Dir Assoc 2007;8:453–7.

[37] Lyles KW, Colon-Emeric C. Treating vitamin D deficiency in long-term care: it should be done yesterday, but how? J Am Med Dir Assoc 2004;5:416–7.

[38] Thomas MK, Lloyd-Jones DM, Thadhani RI, et al. Hypovitaminosis D in medical inpatients. N Engl J Med 1998;338:777–83.

[39] Perry HM 3rd, Horowitz M, Morley JE, et al. Longitudinal changes in serum 25-hydroxyvitamin D in older people. Metabolism 1999;48:1028–32.

[40] Morley JE, Kaiser FE, Perry HM, et al. Longitudinal change in testosterone, luteinizing hormone, and follicle-stimulating hormone in healthy older men. Metab Clin Exper 1997;46:410–3.

[41] Matsumoto AM. Andropause: clinical implications of the decline in serum testosterone levels with aging in men. J Gerontol A Biol Sci Med Sci 2002;57:M76–99.

[42] Morley JE. Androgens and aging. Maturitas 2001;38:61–71.

[43] Morley JE, Kaiser FE, Sih R, et al. Testosterone and frailty. Clin Geriatr Med 1997;13: 685–95.

[44] Dhindsa S, Prabhakar S, Sethi M, et al. Frequent occurrence of hypogonadotropic hypogonadism in type 2 diabetes. J Clin Endocrinol Metab 2004;89:5462–8.

[45] Kalyani RR, Dobs AS. Androgen deficiency, diabetes, and the metabolic syndrome in men. Curr Opin Endocrionl Diabetes Obes 2007;14:226–34.

[46] Mellstrom D, Johnell O, Ljunggren O, et al. Free testosterone is an independent predictor of BMD and prevalent fractures in elderly men: MrOS Sweden. J Bone Miner Res 2006;21: 529–35.

[47] Orwoll E, Lambert LC, Marshall LM, et al. Endogenous testosterone levels, physical performance, and fall risk in older men. Arch Intern Med 2006;166:2124–31.

[48] Sih R, Morley JE, Kaiser FE, et al. Testosterone replacement in older hypogonadal men: a 12-month randomized controlled trial. J Clin Endocrinol Metab 1997;82:1661–7.

[49] Wittert GA, Chapman IM, Haren MT, et al. Oral testosterone supplementation increases muscle and decreases fat mass in healthy elderly males with low-normal gonadal status. J Gerontol A Biol Sci Med Sci 2003;58:618–25.

[50] Page ST, Amory JK, Bowman FD, et al. Exogenous testosterone (T) alone or with finasteride increases physical performance, grip strength, and lean body mass in older men with low serum T. J Clin Endocrinol Metab 2005;90:1502–10.

[51] Morley JE, Perry HM. Androgen deficiency in aging men: role of testosterone replacement therapy. J Lab Clin Med 2000;135:370–8.

[52] Morley JE. Falls and fractures. J Am Med Dir Assoc 2007;8:276–8.

[53] Iwanczyk L, Weintraub NT, Rubenstein LZ. Orthostatic hypotension in the nursing home setting. J Am Med Dir Assoc 2006;7:163–7.

[54] Morley JE. Postprandial hypotension—the ultimate Big Mac attack. J Georntol A Biol Sci Med Sci 2001;56:M741–3.

[55] Edwards BJ, Perry HM 3rd, Kaiser FE, et al. Relationship of age and calcitonin gene-related peptide to postprandial hypotension. Mech Ageing Dev 1996;87:61–73.

[56] Lee A, Patrick P, Wishart J, et al. The effects of miglitol on glucagon-like peptide-1 secretion and appetite sensations in obese type 2 diabetics. Diabetes Obes Metab 2002;4:329–35.

[57] Gentilcore D, Jones KL, O'Donovan DG, et al. Postprandial hypotension—novel insights into pathophysiology and therapeutic implications. Curr Vasc Pharmacol 2006;4:161–71.

[58] Gentilcore D, Bryant B, Wishart JM, et al. Acarbose attenuates the hypotensive response to sucrose and slows gastric emptying in the elderly. Am J Med 2005;118:1289.

[59] Kamel HK, Hussain MS, Tariq S, et al. Failure to diagnose and treat osteoporosis in elderly patients hospitalized with hip fracture. Am J Med 2000;109:326–8.

[60] Harrington JT, Broy SB, Derosa AM, et al. Hip fracture patients are not treated for osteoporosis: a call to action. Arthritis Rheum 2002;47:651–4.

[61] Kamel HK. Update on osteoporosis medications in older nursing facility residents. J Am Med Dir Assoc 2007;8:453–7.

[62] Zarowitz BJ, Stefanacci R, Hollenack K, et al. The application of evidence-based principles of care in older person (issue 1): management of osteoporosis. J Am Med Dir Assoc 2006;7: 102–8.

[63] Drinka PJ, Krause PF, Nest LJ, et al. Determinants of parathyroid hormone levels in nursing home residents. J Am Med Dir Assoc 2007;8:328–31.

[64] Levine JP. Effective strategies to identify postmenopausal women at risk for osteoporosis. Geriatrics 2007;62:22–30.

[65] Dagdelen S, Sener D, Bayraktar M. Influence of type 2 diabetes mellitus on bone mineral density response to bisphosphonates in late postmenopausal osteoporosis. Adv Ther 2007; 24:1314–20.

[66] Rodriguez-Saldana J, Morley JE, Reynoso MT, et al. Diabetes mellitus in a subgroup of older Mexicans: prevalence, associations with cardiovascular risk factors, functional and cognitive impairment, and mortality. J Am Geriatr Soc 2002;50:111–6.

[67] Sakkas GK, Kent-Braun JA, Doyle JW, et al. Effect of diabetes mellitus on muscle size and strength in patients receiving dialysis therapy. Am J Kidney Dis 2006;47:862–9.

[68] Pupim LB, Heimburger O, Qureshi AR, et al. Accelerated lean body mass loss in incident chronic dialysis patients with diabetes mellitus. Kidney Int 2005;68:2368–74.

[69] Dominguez LJ, Barbagallo M. The cardiometabolic syndrome and sarcopenia obesity in older persons. J Cardiometab Syndr 2007;2:183–9.

[70] Sayer AA, Syddall HE, Dennison EM, et al, Hertfordshite Cohort. Grip strength and the metabolic syndrome: findings from the Hertfordshire Cohort. QJM 2007;100:707–13.

[71] Pupim LB, Flakoll PJ, Majchrzak KM, et al. Increased muscle protein breakdown in chronic hemodialysis patients with type 2 diabetes mellitus. Kidney Int 2005;68:1857–65.

[72] Rolland YM, Perry HM 3rd, Patrick P, et al. Loss of appendicular muscle mass and loss of muscle strength in young postmenopausal women. J Gerontol A Biol Sci Med Sci 2007;62: 330–5.

[73] Morley JE, Baumgartner RN, Roubenoff R, et al. Sarcopenia. J Lab Clin Med 2001;137: 231–43.

[74] Waters DL, Baumgartner RN, Garry PJ. Sarcopenia: current perspectives. J Nutr Health Aging 2000;4:133–9.

[75] Janssen I, Heymsfield SB, Ross R. Low relative skeletal muscle mass (sarcopenia) in older persons is associated with functional impairment and physical disability. J Am Geriatr Soc 2002;50:889–96.

[76] Gallagher D, Kuznia P, Heshka S, et al. Adipose tissue in muscle: a novel depot similar in size to visceral adipose tissue. Am J Clin Nutr 2005;81:903–10.

[77] Baumgartner RN, Wayne SJ, Waters DL, et al. Sarcopenic obesity predicts instrumental activities of daily living disability in the elderly. Obes Res 2004;12:1995–2004.

[78] Morley JE. Anorexia, sarcopenia and aging. Nutrition 2001;17:660–3.

[79] Roden M. Muscle triglycerides and mitochondrial function: possible mechanisms for the development of type 2 diabetes. Int J Obes 2005;29(Suppl 2):S111–5.

[80] Casellini CM, Vinik AI. Clinical manifestations and current treatment options for diabetic neuropathies. Endocr Pract 2007;13:550–66.

[81] Guttridge DC. Signaling pathways weigh in on decisions to make or break skeletal muscle. Curr Opin Clin Nutr Metab Care 2004;7:443–50.

[82] Goldspink G. Age-related muscle loss and progressive dysfunction in mechanosensitive growth factor signaling. Ann N Y Acad Sci 2004;1019:294–8.

[83] Dehoux M, van Beneden R, Pasko N, et al. Role of the insulin-like growth factor 1 decline in the induction of atrogin-1/MAFbx during fasting and diabetes. Endocrinology 2004;145: 4806–12.

[84] Kohn FM. Testosterone and body functions. Aging Male 2006;9:183–8.

[85] Haren MT, Malmstrom TK, Banks WA, et al. Lower serum DHEAS levels are associated with a higher degree of physical disability and depressive symptoms in middle-aged to older African American women. Maturitas 2007;57:347–60.

[86] Kim MJ, Morley JE. The hormonal fountains of youth: myth or reality? J Endocrinol Invest 2005;28(11 Suppl Proceedings):5–14.

[87] Lunenfeld B, Nieschlag E. Testosterone therapy in the aging male. Aging Male 2007;10: 139–53.

[88] Kapoor D, Clarke S, Channer KS, et al. Erectile dysfunction is associated with low bioactive testosterone levels and visceral adiposity in men with type 2 diabetes. Int J Androl 2007; 30:500–7.

[89] Kapoor D, Aldred H, Clark S, et al. Clinical and biochemical assessment of hypogonadism in men with type 2 diabetes: correlations with bioavailable testosterone and visceral adiposity. Diabetes Care 2007;30:911–7.

[90] Tsai EC, Matsumoto AM, Fujimoto WY, et al. Association of bioavailable, free, and total testosterone with insulin resistance: influence of sex hormone-binding globulin and body fat. Diabetes Care 2004;27:861–8.

[91] Bhasin S, Taylor WE, Singh R, et al. The mechanisms of androgen effects on body composition: mesenchymal pluripotent cell as the target of androgen action. J Gerontol A Biol Sci Med Sci 2003;58:M1103–10.

[92] Gaskin FS, Farr SA, Banks WA, et al. Ghrelin-induced feeding is dependent on nitric oxide. Peptides 2003;24:913–8.

[93] Diano S, Farr SA, Benoit SC, et al. Ghrelin controls hippocampal spine synapse density and memory performance. Nat Neurosci 2006;9:381–8.

[94] Alonso N, Granada ML, Salinas I, et al. Plasma ghrelin concentrations in type 1 diabetic patients with autoimmune atrophic gastritis. Eur J Endocrinol 2007;157:763–9.

[95] Joulia-Ekaza D, Cabello G. The myostatin gene: physiology and pharmacological relevance. Curr Opin Pharmacol 2007;7:310–5.

[96] Barazzoni R, Zanetti M, Bosutti A, et al. Myostatin expression is not altered by insulin deficiency and replacement in streptozotocin-diabetic rat skeletal muscles. Clin Nutr 2004;23:1413–7.

[97] Morley JE, Baumgartner RN. Cytokine-related aging process. J Gerontol A Biol Sci Med Sci 2004;59:M924–9.

[98] Maggio M, Guralnik JM, Longo DL, et al. Interleukin-6 in aging and chronic disease: a magnificent pathway. J Gerontol A Biol Sci Med Sci 2006;61:575–84.

[99] Cesari M, Penninx BW, Pahor M, et al. Inflammatory markers and physical performance in older persons: the InCHIANTI study. J Gerontol A Biol Sci Med Sci 2004;59:242–8.

[100] Alexandraki K, Piperi C, Kalofoutis C, et al. Inflammatory process in type 2 diabetes: the role of cytokines. Ann N Y Acad Sci 2006;1084:89–117.

[101] Nicola W, Sidhom G, El Khyat Z, et al. Plasma angiotensin II, renin activity and serum angiotensin-converting enzyme activity in non-insulin dependent diabetes mellitus patients with diabetic nephropathy. Endocr J 2001;48:25–31.

[102] Carter CS, Onder G, Kritchevsky SB, et al. Angiotensin-converting enzyme inhibition intervention in elderly persons: effects on body composition and physical performance. J Gerontol A Biol Sci Med Sci 2005;60:1437–46.

[103] Maiese K, Chong ZZ, Shang YC. Mechanistic insights into diabetes mellitus and oxidative stress. Curr Med Chem 2007;14:1729–38.

[104] Candow DG, Chilibeck PD. Effect of creatine supplementation during resistance training on muscle accretion in the elderly. J Nutr Health Aging 2007;11:183–8.

[105] Brose A, Parise G, Tarnopolsky MA. Creatine supplementation enhances isometric strength and body composition improvements following strength exercise training in older adults. J Gerontol A Biol Sci Med Sci 2003;58:11–9.

[106] Thomas DR. Anemia: it's all about quality of life. J Am Med Dir Assoc 2007;8:80–2.

[107] Aoyama L, Weintraub N, Reuben DB. Is weight loss in the nursing home a reversible problem? J Am Med Dir Assoc 2006;7(3 Suppl):S66–72.

[108] Morley JE. Anorexia and weight loss in older persons. J Gerontol A Biol Sci Med Sci 2003; 58:131–7.

[109] Morley JE. Decreased food intake with aging. J Gerontol A Biol Sci Med Sci 2001; 56(Spec 2):81–8.

[110] Morley JE. Anorexia of aging: physiologic and pathologic. Am J Clin Nutr 1997;66:760–73.

[111] Morley JE, Silver AJ. Anorexia in the elderly. Neurobiol Aging 1988;9:9–16.

[112] MacIntosh C, Morley JE, Chapman IM. The anorexia of aging. Nutrition 2000;16:983–95.

[113] Wilson MM, Vaswani S, Liu D, et al. Prevalence and causes of undernutrition in medical outpatients. Am J Med 1998;104:56–63.

[114] Wolfe RR. The underappreciated role of muscle in health and disease. Am J Clin Nutr 2006; 84:475–82.

[115] Schiano V, Brevetti G, Sirico G, et al. Functional status measured by walking impairment questionnaire and cardiovascular risk prediction in peripheral arterial disease: results of the Peripheral Arteriopathy and Cardiovascular Events (PACE) study. Vasc Med 2006;11: 147–54.

[116] McDermott MM, Guralnik JM, Albay M, et al. Impairments of muscles and nerves associated with peripheral arterial disease and their relationship with lower extremity functioning: the InCHIANTI Study. J Am Geriatr Soc 2004;52:405–10.

[117] Landi F, Russo A, Danese P, et al. Anemia status, hemoglobin concentration, and mortality in nursing home older residents. J Am Med Dir Assoc 2007;8:322–7.

[118] Dharmarajan TS, Avula S, Norkus EP. Anemia increases risk for falls in hospitalized older adults: an evaluation of falls in 362 hospitalized, ambulatory, long-term care, and community patients. J Am Med Dir Assoc 2007;8(3 Suppl 2):e9–15.

[119] Steinberg KE. Anemia and falls. J Am Med Dir Assoc 2006;7:327.

[120] Kortebien P, Ferrando A, Lombeida J, et al. Effect of 10 days of bed rest on skeletal muscle in healthy older adults. JAMA 2007;297:1772–4.

[121] Taylor JD. The impact of a supervised strength and aerobic training program on muscular strength and aerobic capacity in individuals with type 2 diabetes. J Strength Cond Res 2007; 21:824–30.

[122] Orr R, de Vos NJ, Singh NA, et al. Power training improves balance in healthy older adults. J Gerontol A Biol Sci Med Sci 2006;61:78–85.

[123] Shumway-Cook A, Silver IF, Lemier M, et al. Effectiveness of a community-based multifactorial intervention on falls and fall risk factors in community-living older adults: a randomized, controlled trial. J Gerontol A Biol Sci Med Sci 2007;62:1420–7.

[124] Latham NK, Bennett DA, Stratton CM, et al. Systematic review of progressive resistance strength training in older adults. J Gerontol A Biol Sci Med Sci 2004;59:48–61.

[125] Joshi S, Morley JE. Cognitive impairment. Med Clin North Am 2006;90:769–87.

[126] Flaherty JH, Rudolph J, Shay K, et al. Delirium is a serious and under-recognized problem: why assessment of mental status should be the sixth vital sign. J Am Med Dir Assoc 2007;8: 273–5.

[127] Morley JE, Flood JF. Psychosocial aspects of diabetes mellitus in older persons. J Am Geriatr Soc 1990;38:605–6.

[128] Mooradian AD, Perryman K, Fitten K, et al. Cortical function in elderly non-insulin dependent diabetic patients. Behavioral and electrophysiologic studies. Arch Intern Med 1988;148:2369–72.

[129] Luchsinger JA, Reitz C, patel B, et al. Relation of diabetes to mild cognitive impairment. Arch Neurol 2007;64:570–5.

[130] Gold SM, Dziobek I, Seat V, et al. Hippocampal damage and memory impairments as possible early brain complications of type 2 diabetes. Diabetologia 2007;50:711–9.

[131] van Harten B, Oosterman J, Muslimovic D, et al. Cognitive impairment and MRI correlates in the elderly patients with type 2 diabetes mellitus. Age Ageing 2007;36:164–70.

[132] Rotkiewicz-Piorun AM, Al Snih S, Raji MA, et al. Cognitive decline in older Mexican Americans with diabetes. J Natl Med Assoc 2006;98:1840–7.

[133] Pasquier F, Boulogne A, Leys D, et al. Diabetes mellitus and dementia. Diabetes Metab 2006;32(5 Pt 1):403–14.

[134] Sun MK, Alkon DL. Links between Alzheimer's disease and diabetes. Drugs Today (Barc) 2006;42:481–9.

[135] Li L, Holscher C. Common pathological processes in Alzheimer disease and type 2 diabetes: a review. Brain Res Rev 2007;56:384–402.

[136] Morley JE, Farr SA, Flood JF. Antibody to amyloid beta protein alleviates impaired acquisition, retention, and memory processing in SAMP8 mice. Neurobiol Learn Mem 2002;78:125–38.

[137] Flood JF, Roberts E, Sherman MA, et al. Topography of a binding site for small amnestic peptides deduced from structure-activity studies: relation to amnestic effect of amyloid beta protein. Proc Natl Acad Sci USA 1994;91:380–4.

[138] Flood JF, Morley JE, Roberts E. Amnestic effects in mice of four synthetic peptides homologous to amyloid beta protein from patients with Alzheimer disease. Proc Natl Acad Sci USA 1991;88:3363–6.

[139] Li C, Ford ES, Strine TW, et al. Prevalence of depression among U.S. adults with diabetes: findings from the 2006 behavioral risk factor surveillance system. Diabetes Care 2008;31:105–7.

[140] Rosenthal MJ, Fajardo M, Gilmore S, et al. Hospitalization and mortality of diabetes in older adults—1 3-year prospective study. Diabetes Care 1998;21:231–5.

[141] Morley JE. Diabetes mellitus: a major disease of older persons. J Gerontol A Biol Sci Med Sci 2000;55:M255–6.

[142] Cabrera MA, Mesas AE, Garcia AR, et al. Malnutrition and depression among community-dwelling elderly people. J Am Med Dir Assoc 2007;8:582–4.

[143] Tariq SH, Tumosa N, Chibnall JT, et al. Comparison of the Saint Louis University mental status examination and the mini-mental state examination for detecting dementia and mild neurocognitive disorder—a pilot study. Am J Geriatr Psychiatry 2006;14:900–10.

[144] Banks WA, Morley JE. Memories are made of this: recent advances in understanding cognitive impairments and dementia. J Gerontol A Biol Sci Med Sci 2003;58:314–21.

[145] Lee J, Monette J, Sourial N, et al. The use of a cholinesterase inhibitor review committee in long-term care. J Am Med Dir Assoc 2007;8:243–7.

[146] Christensen MD, White HK. Dementia assessment and management. J Am Med Dir Assoc 2007;8(3 Suppl 2):e89–98.

[147] Standridge JB. Current status and future promise of pharmacotherapeutic strategies for Alzheimer's disease. J Am Med Dir Assoc 2006;7(3 Suppl):S46–51.

[148] Belgeri M, Morley JE. A step back in time: is there a place for older drugs in the treatment of dementia? J Georntol A Biol Sci Med Sci 2004;59:1025–8.

[149] Poon HF, Farr SA, Thongboonkerd V, et al. Proteomic analysis of specific brain proteins in aged SAMP8 mice treated with alpha-lipoic acid: implications for aging and age-related neurodegenerative disorders. Neurochem Int 2005;46:159–68.

[150] Farr SA, Poon HF, Dogrukol-Ak D, et al. The antioxidants alpha-lipoic acid and N-acetylcysteine reverse memory impairment and brain oxidative stress in aged SAMP8 mice. J Neurochem 2003;84:1173–83.

ELSEVIER
SAUNDERS

CLINICS IN
GERIATRIC
MEDICINE

Clin Geriatr Med 24 (2008) 471–487

Hyperlipidemia in the Elderly

Nicole Ducharme, DO*, Rani Radhamma, MD

Division of Endocrinology, Saint Louis University Medical Center, 1402 South Grand Boulevard, Donco Building, 2nd Floor, St. Louis, MO 63104, USA

People are now living longer, largely because of a combination of falling rates of fertility and mortality, thus producing a greater proportion of older people in society [1]. Thirty times more centenarians were alive in 2000 than in 1900, and the population growth in the elderly segment of society is expected to continue at an exponential rate. Vascular disease is responsible for more than a quarter of all deaths worldwide. More than 80% of individuals who die of coronary heart disease (CHD) are older than 65 years. Although a myocardial infarction may be perceived as fatal, heart attacks do not always lead to death but to conditions such as congestive heart failure, ischemic cardiomyopathy, and angina, which greatly impact quality of life. These issues are only a few that must be contemplated when considering the clinical and economic effects of preventive therapies in the elderly population.

Despite the high prevalence of heart disease and stroke in the elderly population, whether predictors of these conditions during middle age remain clinically relevant as age increases is still unclear. Cholesterol, for example, is a well-defined independent risk factor for premature death in middle-aged individuals, and apparently does not have the same predictive power in older patients. Over the past 40 years, a substantial amount of research has established the importance of lipids and lipoproteins as risk factors for developing cardiovascular disease. Elevated plasma levels of total and low-density lipoprotein (LDL) cholesterol are associated with increased risk, whereas the plasma high-density lipoprotein (HDL) cholesterol level is inversely related to risk for CHD.

No evidence shows that coronary artery disease is fundamentally different in older compared with younger patients [2]. Atherosclerosis continues to progress into the elderly years, and older people have much more

---

* Corresponding author.
E-mail address: nducharme3@hotmail.com (N. Ducharme).

0749-0690/08/$ - see front matter © 2008 Elsevier Inc. All rights reserved.
doi:10.1016/j.cger.2008.03.007   *geriatric.theclinics.com*

coronary atherosclerosis than those who are middle-aged. Rates of athero-genesis vary greatly and depend on the presence or absence of risk factors. Two thirds to three quarters of individuals older than 65 years have either clinical CHD or subclinical atherosclerotic disease. Thus, risk reduction in these patients is essential.

The lipid hypothesis states that an elevated plasma cholesterol level is casually associated with cardiovascular disease, and that lowering it will reduce risk for disease. This hypothesis was tested in a series of early trials, mainly using bile acid sequestrants and fibric acid derivatives.

Although the results partially supported the notion that lowering choles-terol was beneficial in terms of reducing cardiovascular risk, overall safety was a concern [1]. However, these concerns were dispelled when a new gen-eration of lipid-lowering drugs was developed.

HMG-CoA reductase inhibitors, otherwise known as statin drugs, were introduced in the 1980s and used to test the lipid hypothesis in a series of landmark trials. Although no published statin trial has been directed exclu-sively at elderly subjects, elderly cohorts have been included in several stud-ies, which have shown that older individuals seem to experience similar benefit from statin therapy as younger patients.

Hyperlipidemia in the elderly

Hyperlipidemia refers to elevated levels of lipids in the blood. Lipids, such as cholesterol and triglycerides, are insoluble in plasma. Circulating lipid is carried in lipoproteins that transport the lipid to various tissues for energy use, lipid deposition, steroid hormone production, and bile acid formation. The lipoprotein consists of esterified and unesterified cho-lesterol, triglycerides, phospholipids, and protein. Most people who have hyperlipidemia experience no symptoms.

Abnormalities in lipoprotein metabolism are a major predisposing factor to atherosclerosis, increasing risk for CHD. CHD is the leading cause of morbidity and mortality in the elderly population [2]. Approximately 80% of all deaths caused by CHD occur in this age group. Almost 25% of men and 42% of women older than 65 years have abnormal serum total cho-lesterol level greater than 240 mg/dL [3]. At menopause, LDL cholesterol increases substantially because of declining estrogen levels and weight gain [4]. The potential for treatment benefit within this population is high. As lipid levels decrease, so does the risk for developing CHD and experienc-ing a stroke.

Age-related changes in lipoprotein metabolism

Total cholesterol levels increase in men after the onset of puberty until 50 years of age, followed by a plateau until 70 years of age. Serum cholesterol concentration then declines slightly. The most important factor influencing cholesterol may be weight change [5].

In women, the serum cholesterol concentration is slightly higher than in men before 20 to 25 years of age. Between 25 to 55 years of age, the serum cholesterol increases, although at a slower incremental rate than in men. Cholesterol levels in women are equal to those of men between 55 and 60 years of age, and exceed those of men in older age groups.

The age-related changes in the serum cholesterol concentration primarily result from an increase in LDL cholesterol [6]. However, HDL cholesterol levels do not vary much with age, and are approximately 10 mg/dL higher in women than men.

Classification

Five major lipoproteins exist, each with a different function: chylomicrons, very–low-density lipoproteins (VLDLs), intermediate-density lipoproteins (IDLs), LDLs, and HDLs. The protein components of the lipoprotein are known as apolipoproteins or apoproteins. The different apolipoproteins serve as cofactors for enzymes, and ligands for receptors. Defects in apolipoprotein metabolism lead to abnormalities in lipid handling [7].

Chylomicrons

Chylomicrons are very large particles that carry dictary lipid. They are associated with various apolipoproteins, including A-I, A-II, A-IV, B-48, C-I, C-II, C-III, and E.

Very–low-density lipoprotein

VLDL has endogenous triglycerides and, to a lesser degree, cholesterol. The major apolipoproteins associated with VLDL are B-100, C-I, C-II, C-III, and E.

Intermediate-density lipoprotein

IDL has cholesterol esters and triglycerides. It is associated with apolipoproteins B-100, C-III, and E.

Low-density lipoprotein

LDL carries cholesterol esters and is associated with apolipoprotein B-100.

High-density lipoprotein

HDL also carries cholesterol esters, and is associated with apolipoproteins A-I, A-II, C-I, C-II, C-III, D, and E.

Clinical classification of dyslipidemias

The major classes of dyslipidemia are classified according to the Fredrickson phenotype [8]:

- Fredrickson phenotype I: serum concentration of chylomicrons elevated; triglycerides concentrations are elevated to higher than the 99th percentile
- Fredrickson phenotype IIa: serum concentration of LDL cholesterol elevated; the total cholesterol concentration is higher than the 90th percentile. Concentrations of triglyceride and/or apolipoprotein B may also be 90th percentile
- Fredrickson phenotype IIb: serum concentrations of LDL and VLDL cholesterol elevated; total cholesterol and/or triglycerides may be 90th percentile and apolipoprotein B 90th percentile
- Fredrickson phenotype III: serum concentration of VLDL remnants and chylomicrons elevated; total cholesterol and triglycerides higher than the 90th percentile
- Fredrickson phenotype IV: serum concentrations of VLDL elevated; total cholesterol may be higher than the 90th percentile and may also see triglyceride concentrations higher than the 90th percentile or low HDL
- Fredrickson phenotype V: elevated serum concentrations of chylomicrons and VLDL; triglycerides higher than the 99th percentile

Total cholesterol

An elevated total cholesterol level is associated with an increased risk for CHD. A desirable total cholesterol level is usually less than 200 mg/dL. A total cholesterol level of 200 to 239 mg/dL is borderline high, whereas a value of 240 mg/dL or more is high. However, most decisions about treatment are made based on the level of LDL or HDL rather than total cholesterol. Total cholesterol can be measured any time of day; individuals do not need to fast before testing.

Low-density lipoprotein cholesterol

LDL cholesterol is a more accurate predictor of CHD than total cholesterol. Higher LDL cholesterol concentrations are associated with an increased incidence of CHD.

Triglycerides

Hypertriglyceridemia is associated with an increased risk for cardiovascular disease [9]. Triglycerides are atherogenic because they are rich in apolipoprotein C-III, which delays the lipolysis of VLDL and inhibits its uptake and clearance from plasma. Hypertriglyceridemia can also promote athero-thrombosis through increasing coagulability and blood viscosity [10]. Hypertriglyceridemia tends to be associated with low HDL levels [11,12]. Triglyceride concentrations are stratified as follows:

- Normal: less than 150 mg/dL
- Borderline high: 150 to 199 mg/dL
- High: 200 to 499 mg/dL
- Very high: greater than 500 mg/dL

Triglycerides should be measured after fasting for 12 to 14 hours.

High-density lipoprotein cholesterol

An inverse relationship exists between plasma HDL cholesterol levels and cardiovascular risk. HDL, in contrast to LDL and VLDL, has antiathero-genic properties that include reverse cholesterol transport, maintenance of endothelial function, protection against thrombosis, and maintenance of low blood viscosity through a permissive action on red cell deformability. Values greater than 75 mg/dL are associated with a longevity syndrome. Similar to total cholesterol, HDL cholesterol can be measured on any blood specimen. Patients do not need to be fasting.

Non–high-density lipoprotein cholesterol

Non-HDL cholesterol is defined as the difference between the total and HDL cholesterol. It includes all cholesterol in lipoprotein particles that is considered atherogenic, including LDL, lipoprotein, intermediate-density lipoprotein, and VLDL. It has been suggested that the non-HDL cholesterol fraction may be a better tool for risk assessment than LDL cholesterol.

Pathways of lipid metabolism

Three main pathways are responsible for the generation and transport of lipids within the body: exogenous, endogenous, and reverse cholesterol transport.

Exogenous pathway

After digestion and absorption of dietary fat, free fatty acids combine with glycerol to form triglycerides, and cholesterol is esterified by acyl-coen-zyme A: cholesterol acyltransferase (ACAT) to form cholesterol esters. Triglycerides and cholesterol are assembled intracellularly as chylomicrons. In the blood, circulating chylomicrons interact at the capillaries of adipose tissue and muscle cells, releasing triglycerides to the adipose tissue to be stored and available for the body's energy needs. The enzyme lipoprotein lipase (LPL) hydrolyzes the triglycerides, and free-fatty acids are released. Some of the components of the chylomicrons are "repackaged" into other lipoproteins;, for example, some apolipoproteins are transferred to HDL, and the remaining chylomicron remnant particles are removed from the plasma by way of chylomicron remnant receptors present on the liver.

Endogenous pathway

The endogenous pathway involves the liver-synthesizing lipoproteins. Triglycerides and cholesterol ester are generated by the liver, packaged into VLDL particles, and released into the circulation. VLDL is then hydrolyzed by LPL in tissues to release fatty acids and glycerol. The fatty acids are taken up by muscle cells for energy or by adipose cells for storage. Once processed by LPL, the VLDL becomes a VLDL remnant. Most VLDL remnants are taken up by the liver by way of the LDL receptor, and the remaining remnant particles become IDL, a smaller, denser lipoprotein than VLDL. Some IDL particles are reabsorbed by the liver through the LDL receptor, whereas others are hydrolyzed in the liver by hepatic triglyceride lipase to form LDL, a smaller, denser particle than IDL.

LDL is the main carrier of circulating cholesterol within the body. It is used by extrahepatic cells for cell membrane and steroid hormone synthesis. Most LDL particles are taken up by LDL receptors in the liver, and the remaining particles are removed by way of scavenger pathways at the cellular level.

Once the LDL is taken up by receptors, free cholesterol is released and accumulates within the cells. LDL receptor activity and uptake regulates plasma LDL concentration through several mechanisms, including decreasing the synthesis of HMG-CoA reductase, the enzyme that controls the rate of de novo cholesterol synthesis by the cell. This process suppresses the synthesis of new LDL receptors in the cells and activates the enzyme acylcoenzyme A cholesterol acyltransferase, which esterifies free cholesterol into cholesterol ester, storing cholesterol in the cell.

Reverse cholesterol transport

Reverse cholesterol transport is the process through which cholesterol is removed from the tissues and returned to the liver. HDL is the key lipoprotein involved in reverse cholesterol transport and the transfer of cholesteryl esters between lipoproteins. The smallest and most dense lipoprotein particle, HDL is formed through a maturation process whereby precursor particles (nascent HDL) secreted by the liver and intestine proceed through a series of conversions known as the *HDL cycle* to attract cholesterol from cell membranes and free cholesterol to the core of the HDL particle.

The exact mechanism is not well understood, but several mechanisms have been suggested, including the action of cholesteryl ester transfer protein, which transforms HDL into a triglyceride-rich particle that inter-acts with hepatic triglyceride lipase. Cholesterol ester–rich HDL may also be taken up directly by the receptors in the liver. Another mechanism may be that cholesterol esters are delivered directly to the liver for uptake without catabolism of the HDL cholesterol particle.

The net effect is the removal of excess cholesterol from cells, which constitutes most of the antiatherogenic effect of HDL.

Lipoproteins and atherosclerosis

Mechanisms of increased atherogenecity are believed to be related to two effects-endothelial dysfunction which is independent of the concentration of lipoproteins and direct effect of lipoproteins. The direct effect includes enhanced oxidative susceptibility [13,14] and reduced clearance by LDL receptors in the liver with increased LDL receptor-independent binding in the arterial wall [15,16]. Small dense LDL is indirectly associated with atherogenic risk through it's inverse relationship with HDL cholesterol, functions as a marker for accumulation of atherogenic triglyceride remnant particles, and plays a role in insulin resistance [17].

LDL cholesterol promotes inflammatory and immune changes through cytokine release from macrophages and antibody production. Release of cy-tokines stimulates smooth muscle proliferation. Thus, foam cell and platelet accumulation and smooth muscle proliferation contribute to the formation of an atherosclerotic plaque.

Cholesterol screening guidelines

The United States Preventive Services Task Force provides several recommendations for cholesterol screening.

- Lipid screening should begin at 35 years of age in men and 45 years in women. Those at risk for CHD should be treated for abnormal lipid levels.
- Screening is recommended for men aged 20 to 35 years and women aged 20 to 45 years who have diabetes; a family history of cardiovascular dis-ease before age 50 years in male relatives or 60 years in female relatives; a family history of familial hyperlipidemia; or multiple CHD risk factors (eg, tobacco use, hypertension).
- Screening should include total cholesterol and HDL cholesterol levels, and can be measured in nonfasting or fasting samples.
- The optimal interval between screenings is uncertain; reasonable options include every 5 years, with shorter intervals for those who have high-normal lipid levels, and longer intervals for low-risk individuals who have low or normal levels.

- The age to stop screening is not established.
- Screening may be appropriate in older people who have never undergone screening, but repeated screening is less important in older people because lipid levels are less likely to increase after 65 years of age.

Benefits of managing hyperlipidemia

The causal link between elevated LDL cholesterol and CHD is now firmly established [18]. Compelling evidence also supports an independent link between low HDL cholesterol levels and high triglyceride levels and atherosclerosis.

In the Multiple Risk Factor Intervention Trial, CHD rates declined progressively with lower total cholesterol levels down to a level of 150 mg/dL, corresponding to an LDL cholesterol level of approximately 100 mg/dL. Drug treatment with statins for a mean duration of 5.4 years was associated with a 20% reduction in total cholesterol, 28% reduction in LDL cholesterol, 13% reduction in triglycerides and 5% increase in HDL cholesterol. Statin therapy also led to a 31% reduction in major coronary events and a 21% reduction in all-cause mortality. The reduction of major coronary events was similar for both men and women and between individuals aged 65 years or older and those younger than 65 years (32% and 31%, respectively).

The Framingham Study provided the best data correlating low HDL cholesterol levels with an independent CHD event risk. Results showed that every 4 mg/dL decrease in HDL cholesterol level was associated with an approximate 10% increase in CHD risk. Low HDL cholesterol levels have been found to be an even more important predictor of risk, especially when accompanied by elevated triglyceride and high LDL cholesterol levels.

Elevated triglyceride levels have more recently become recognized as an independent predictor of CHD risk. The largest risk assessment of elevated triglyceride levels came from a meta-analysis of 17 studies and found that for every 88 mg/dL increase in triglyceride level, the relative risk for CHD increased 14% in men and 37% in women after adjusting for HDL cholesterol levels. Hence, elevated triglycerides alone increase the risk for CHD. However, when high triglycerides are associated with other metabolic derangements, such as increased waist circumference, hypertension, hypercoagulable state, small dense LDL cholesterol, low HDL cholesterol, and insulin resistance, the risk for developing coronary thrombosis increases significantly.

Guidelines for the treatment of dyslipidemia

The National Cholesterol Education Program Adult Treatment Panel II (NCEP ATP-II), published in 1993, recommends using CHD risk status as a guide to therapy intensity [19]. NCEP ATP-II identifies LDL cholesterol as the primary target of lipid-lowering therapy. Although lower LDL cholesterol levels show a definite trend toward decreased total mortality in patients who have CHD, no clinical trial or meta-analysis has shown a reduction in total mortality in patients who have no established CHD (primary prevention).

In 2001, The Adult Treatment Panel III (ATP III) issued new evidence-based treatment guidelines (Table 1). These guidelines introduced a new secondary target of therapy, namely non–HDL cholesterol, in patients who have elevated triglycerides (≥ 200 mg/dL) [20]. Non–HDL cholesterol equates to VLDL + LDL cholesterol (which when calculated, includes IDLs). The non–HDL cholesterol goal is 30 mg/dL higher than the target LDL cholesterol goal.

Non–HDL cholesterol was added as a secondary target of therapy to account for the atherogenic potential associated with remnant lipoproteins in patients who have hypertriglyceridemia. Because statins lower LDL cholesterol and non–HDL cholesterol to a similar percentage, recent clinical trials do not differentiate between these lipid measures regarding their relative benefits in risk reduction (Table 2).

Primary prevention

Because most first CHD events occur after 65 years of age, primary prevention in the elderly is a topic of great importance [2]. The NCEP emphasizes that the optimal approach is lifetime prevention, with the goal of reducing the total burden of coronary atherosclerosis in the population. To sustain lifetime prevention efforts, older persons should be encouraged to have healthy eating habits, exercise regularly, and eliminate excess body weight, which will improve health and reduce elevated serum cholesterol.

Table 1
Approach to the management of hyperlipidemia

Category	Risk factors[b]	LDL goal	Initiate lifestyle change[a]	Consider drug therapy
Very high risk	Established coronary artery disease plus one of the risk factors[c]	<70 mg/dL	≥70 mg/dL	≥70 mg/dL
High	CHD or CHD equivalent	<100 mg/dL	≥100 mg/dL	≥100 mg/dL
Moderate	≥2	<130 mg/dL	≥130 mg/dL	≥160 mg/dL
Low	0–1	<160 mg/dL	≥160 mg/dL	≥190 mg/dL

[a] Lifestyle changes (eg, smoking cessation, weight loss, exercise) should be recommended for a minimum of 3 to 6 months. However, drug therapy may be considered in 4 to 6 weeks if the patient is not approaching LDL cholesterol goal, especially those who are elderly.

[b] Risk factors include cigarette smoking, low HDL cholesterol, age (≥ 45 years in men, ≥ 55 years in women), family history, and hypertension.

[c] Multiple major risk factors (especially diabetes), severe and poorly controlled risk factors (especially continued cigarette smoking), multiple risk factors of the metabolic syndrome (especially triglycerides >200 mg/dL plus non–HDL cholesterol ≥ 130 mg/dL with low HDL cholesterol <40 mg/dL), or acute coronary syndromes based on the Pravastatin or Atorvastatin Evaluation and Infection Therapy and Infection Therapy study.

Table 2
Target lipid levels for treatment

Lipid parameter	Target level
Total cholesterol	<200 mg/dL
Triglycerides	<150 mg/dL
LDL	Risk factor dependent, but <100 mg/dL in those who have diabetes mellitus, coronary artery disease, or peripheral vascular disease
HDL	>40 mg/dL in men, > 50 mg/dL in women
Non-HDL	30 mg/dL higher than the LDL cholesterol goal

Two primary prevention trials using statins included a large number of older people: The Air Force/Texas Coronary Atherosclerosis Prevention Study (AFCAPS) and the West of Scotland Coronary Prevention Study (WOSCOPS). AFCAPS included 6605 participants, including 1416 men and women who were aged 65 years or older [21]. This study showed a 37% reduction in major coronary events among the whole group, and similar results were observed in the older group, suggesting that primary prevention with statin therapy is beneficial in the young elderly, up to 75 years of age, without significant adverse effects.

Based on this study, the Committee of National Cholesterol Education Program published an article suggesting that drug therapy be considered for primary prevention in elderly individuals who have significant hypercholesterolemia, based on (1) general health status and functional capacity, and (2) CHD risk stratification. According to these guidelines, drug therapy should be considered in elderly patients who have no debilitating diseases and a very high LDL cholesterol of 190 mg/dL or higher, or in those who have an LDL cholesterol level of 160 to 189 mg/dL and two or more CHD risk factors.

In the West of Scotland Coronary Prevention Study, 6595 men aged 45 to 64 years who had no heart disease and hypercholesterolemia were randomized to treatment with pravastatin, 40 mg daily, or placebo [22]. Pravastatin therapy was associated with a 25% reduction in serum LDL chemotherapy, and showed a 29% reduction in major coronary events and 23% decrease in total mortality after 5 years of treatment.

The Cardiovascular Health Study, a cohort study of 1250 women and 664 men older than 65 years who had hypercholesterolemia requiring treatment, also showed statin treatment to be beneficial for primary prevention [23]. In this report, statin use was associated with significantly decreased risk for cardiovascular events and all-cause mortality.

Finally, the Anglo-Scandinavian Cardiac Outcomes Trial-Lipid Lowering Arm (ASCOT-LLA) Trial, which randomized 19,342 patients who had hypertension to atorvastatin (10 mg) or placebo over 3.3 years, showed that atorvastatin lowered nonfatal myocardial infarction by 36% and decreased total cardiovascular events by 21% compared with placebo [24].

The position paper from the Society of Geriatric Cardiology recommends lipid-lowering agents for individuals aged 65 to 80 years who do not have coronary artery disease with a serum total cholesterol level of 240 mg/dL or higher, or serum LDL cholesterol level of 160 mg/dL or higher, and one other major risk factor such as hypertension, diabetes mellitus, smoking, or a serum HDL cholesterol level less than 35 mg/dL, despite diet. This treatment is intended to reduce the serum total cholesterol to less than 200 mg/dL and the serum LDL cholesterol to less than 130 mg/dL [25]. Reasonable treatment for high-risk persons older than 80 years who have hypercholesterolemia and no coronary artery disease, who are otherwise healthy, includes diet and lipid-lowering agents.

Secondary prevention

Multiple prospective clinical trials have shown the benefits of lipid-lowering therapy on total mortality, coronary events, coronary artery procedures, and stroke in patients who have established CHD [26]. These trials, however, included few elderly participants, creating some uncertainty about the benefits of these agents in the older population.

Most data on the effect of statins on preventing CHD in the elderly are derived from secondary prevention trials. Three large secondary prevention trials using statin agents have been performed: the Scandinavian Simvastatin Survival Study (4S), Cholesterol and Recurrent Events (CARE) trial, and Long-Term Intervention with Pravastatin in Ischemic Disease (LIPID) study [2].

The 4S trial compared simvastatin (20–40 mg) with placebo and showed that, compared with placebo, it decreased total mortality by 35% and coronary mortality by 42% in both sexes and individuals aged 60 years or older over 5 years [22].

The CARE trial evaluated the effect of pravastatin on coronary events after myocardial infarction in patients who had total cholesterol less than 240 mg/dL. Subjects were randomized to pravastatin, 40 mg, or placebo [27]. This study showed that pravastatin lowered total cholesterol by 20% and LDL cholesterol levels by 32% over a 5-year follow-up. Patients treated with pravastatin also showed a 24% lower incidence of fatal CHD, confirmed myocardial infarction, and a reduced rate of coronary artery bypass surgery or percutaneous transluminal coronary angioplasty.

The LIPID study evaluated the use of pravastatin in 9014 patients aged 31 to 75 years (36% of patients ≥ 65 years of age) who had a history of myocardial infarction or unstable angina and serum cholesterol levels of 155 to 271 mg/dL [22]. During the 6-year follow-up, patients treated with pravastatin had a 22% reduction in overall mortality, 29% reduction in risk for myocardial infarction, 24% reduction in risk for CHD or nonfatal myocardial infarction, and 20% reduction in risk for coronary revascularization.

However, the Prospective Study of Pravastatin in the Elderly at Risk (PROSPER) study was the first to evaluate significantly older patients and to include mostly women (52%). This study randomized patients aged 70 to 82 years who had a history of risk factors for vascular disease to treatment with pravastatin, 40 mg/d, or placebo [28]. During a mean follow-up of 3 years, pravastatin was found to lower LDL cholesterol levels by 34% and triglycerides by 13%, and reduce risk for coronary death, nonfatal myocardial infarction, and stroke by 15%. However, it failed to reduce total mortality or improve function or cognitive dysfunction.

Statin drug treatment

Meta-analysis

A meta-analysis of five randomized trials, two primary (West of Scottland Coronary Prevention Study, Airforce/Texas Coronary Atherosclerosis Prevention Study) and three secondary (4S, CARE, LIPID), estimated the risk reduction of CHD and total mortality associated with statin drug treatment, particularly in the elderly. Results showed that active treatment was associated with a 34% risk reduction in major coronary events in the two primary prevention trials and a 30% risk reduction in the three secondary prevention trials [29]. Active treatment was associated with a lower risk for coronary disease mortality, cardiovascular mortality, and all-cause mortality compared with controls [29]. This finding was confirmed in another meta-analysis comparing individuals >60 years of age [30].

Dosage

In the elderly, the dosage of any cholesterol-lowering medication should be started at a low dose to avoid adverse events, and then titrated slowly to achieve optimal LDL cholesterol levels. This method should be used when initiating any antihyperlipidemic agent, including fibrates, Niaspan, or bile acid sequestrants, and a combination of agents must be initiated with caution because it increases risk for side effects.

The studies mentioned earlier have shown that, compared with placebo, statin therapy reduces cardiovascular morbidity and mortality. However, no studies assessed intensive therapy compared with moderate therapy in older individuals until the Study Assessing Goals in the Elderly (SAGE) study was conducted. This study looked at 893 patients between ages 65 and 85 years who had coronary artery disease who were randomized to atorvastatin, 80 mg/d, or pravastatin, 40 mg/d [31]. This study showed that, compared with moderate pravastatin therapy, intensive atorvastatin therapy was associated with reductions in cholesterol, major acute cardiovascular events, and death, in addition to the reductions in ischemia seen with both therapies.

Based on this study, intensive therapy seems to have better outcome; however, in the elderly population, risks versus benefits must still be considered and dosages titrated to avoid adverse reactions. Despite this data, patients should be maintained on the lowest dose needed to achieve desired LDL cholesterol levels.

Adverse effects

Elevation of serum hepatic transaminases higher than three times the upper limit of normal occurs in approximately 1% of persons taking statins [21]. This increase is usually reversible and rarely causes clinical significance. Skeletal muscle myopathy occurs in fewer than 0.2% of persons taking statins. The risk for skeletal muscle myopathy is higher if statins are used in combination with gemfibrozil, nicotinic acid, erythromycin, or cyclosporine A. Statin drugs should not be used in persons who have active liver disease or unexplained persistent elevated serum hepatic transaminases (Table 3).

Monitoring

Liver function tests should be obtained before initiating therapy, at 6 and 12 weeks after initiating therapy, after increasing the drug dose, and at 6-month intervals [21]. Lipid profiles should be checked 4 or more weeks after a statin is initiated or a dosage adjustment occurs.

Ezetimibe

Although statins are the most effective drugs for treating hypercholesterolemia [32], many elderly patients are cannot achieve optimal LDL cholesterol levels with statins alone, because increasing dose heightens the risk for adverse reactions, with myopathy the most common. Therefore, alternative treatment with other antihyperlipidemic agents, such as ezetimibe, may be necessary.

Ezetimibe is a cholesterol absorption inhibitor that prevents intestinal absorption of dietary and biliary cholesterol without affecting the absorption of triglycerides or fat-soluble vitamins. In addition, like HMG-CoA reductase inhibitors, ezetimibe inhibits cholesterol synthesis in the liver, and therefore, when coadministered with different statins, has been shown to produce greater LDL cholesterol reductions. It has also been shown to have more favorable effects on other lipid parameters, including apolipoprotein B, non–HDL cholesterol, triglycerides, and HDL cholesterol, than statin monotherapy.

Table 3
Effects of drugs used to treat hyperlipidemia

Medication	LDL	HDL	Triglycerides	Major side effects
HMG-CoA inhibitors (statins)	↓↓↓	↑	↓	Myopathy hepatotoxicity
Bile acid sequestrants	↓↓	—	↑	Constipation, flatulence
Fibrates	↑	↑↑	↓↓↓	Hepatotoxicity gallstones
Niaspan	↓	↑↑↑	↓↓	Flushing, worsened peptic ulcer disease, hyperglycemia, hepatotoxicity

Abbreviations: ↓, low; ↑, high.

One study compared the efficacy and safety of statin monotherapy (lovastatin or pravastatin, 10, 20, or 40 mg; simvastatin or atorvastatin, 10, 20, 40, or 80 mg) with ezetimibe, 10 mg, plus a statin in older and younger adults who had primary hypercholesterolemia [33]. This study found that coadministering ezetimibe and statin produced significant incremental reductions in LDL cholesterol compared with statin monotherapy. The beneficial effects on LDL cholesterol, triglycerides, and HDL cholesterol were similar among older and younger patients who had hypercholesterolemia, with a favorable safety profile across all age groups. However, a recent press announcement suggested that adding ezetimibe to a statin produced no advantage.

Compliance

Data suggest that elderly individuals are less likely to receive lipid-lowering medications or adhere to statin therapy [26]. Mendelson and Aronow [34] reviewed the charts of 1492 older patients (mean age $\pm$ SD, 80 ± 8 years) seen in a primary care outpatient geriatric practice who had no contraindications to lipid-lowering drug therapy [34]. Among 391 patients who had a documented history of myocardial infarction and an LDL cholesterol level greater than 125 mg/dL, lipid-lowering agents were prescribed for 53% of patients younger than 70 years, 54% of patients aged 70 to 80 years, and 47% of patients older than 80 years, suggesting that lipid-lowering therapy was prescribed appropriately for approximately only half of the patients.

Landmark clinical trials have shown survival benefits for statins, which usually begin after 1 to 2 years of treatment [35]. A study was designed to compare 2-year adherence after statin initiation in three cohorts of patients: those who had recent acute coronary syndrome, those who had chronic coronary artery disease, and those who did not have coronary disease (primary prevention). All patients in the study were 66 years of age or older, had received at least one statin prescription between January 1994 and December 1998 and did not have a statin prescription in the prior year, and were followed up for 2 years from their first statin prescription. The acute coronary syndrome group enrolled 22,379 patients, the chronic coronary artery disease group had 36,106, and the primary prevention group had 85,020. Adherence was defined as a statin being dispensed at least every 120 days after the index prescription for 2 years.

This study showed that simvastatin was the most frequently prescribed statin (30.1%), followed closely by atorvastatin (29.0) and pravastatin (25.4%), with relatively little use of lovastatin (9.6%), fluvastatin (3.8%), and cerivastatin (2.0%). Adherence continually diminished from initiation of therapy through 2 years follow-up in a progressive manner, with at least 25% of patients discontinuing statin therapy by 6 months in all groups.

Another retrospective cohort study evaluating persistent use of statins in the elderly, included 34,501 patients who were 65 years of age or older and had a statin initiated between 1990 and 1998. Patients were followed up until death, disenrollment, or December 31, 1999 [36]. This study also showed that statin therapy in older patients declines substantially over time, with the greatest drop occurring in the first 6 months of treatment. In this study, nonadherent patients comprised 29% of the population at 6 months and 56% at 60 months. This study seems to show that patients who were non-white, Medicaid recipients, 75 years of age or older, and being treated for depression were more likely to have suboptimal compliance.

Several reasons exist as to why patients may be noncompliant, including cost, adverse effects, coronary events despite being on lipid-lowering agents, and the perception that the drug is not beneficial. Therefore, improving patient understanding of cardiovascular risk, the medication regimen, and potential benefits of persistence with statin therapy may further enhance compliance. However, further investigation into improving compliance is needed in clinical trials.

Summary

Primary and secondary prevention trials have conclusively shown that lowering serum cholesterol levels reduces morbidity and mortality from CHD [22]. However, the major limitation of these studies is that they included young elderly patients, up to age 75 years. Therefore, conclusions regarding the impact of lowering cholesterol among elderly individuals are based primarily on the known pathophysiologic role of hypercholesterol-emia in the atherosclerotic process, and extrapolation from results in elderly subgroups within larger trials [1].

Collectively, published data indicate that elderly individuals are a high-risk group who would benefit significantly from lipid-lowering statin therapy to reduce cardiovascular morbidity and mortality [1]. Nevertheless, a long-standing trend exists toward underdiagnosis and treatment of hyper-cholesterolemia in the elderly [22], illustrated in a prospective study of 500 patients who had a mean age of 81 years and a Q-wave myocardial infarc-tion. Although 67% had an LDL cholesterol concentration higher than 125 mg/dL, only 5% were treated with lipid-lowering drugs. Several other studies have documented similar findings. Hence, health care professionals must continue to be aggressive in screening and treating patients, targeting cholesterol levels, despite their age.

Cholesterol screening and treatment in the elderly population is benefi-cial. However, no set guidelines exist on which patients are good candidates, and this remains an area of controversy. Therefore, determining whether to treat high cholesterol in the elderly must be individualized, based on the patient's biologic age, comorbidities, expected lifespan, quality of life, and risks versus benefits.

In addition, regardless of age, dietary and lifestyle changes are the foun-dation for successful clinical management of hyperlipidemia. Drug therapy should be added only when patients do not achieve target lipid levels with dietary therapy within 6 months, or when the short-term risk of future CHD events is sufficiently high to embark on prompt lipid lowering [18]. Although these concepts are mainstream in endocrinology and cardiology, many geriatricians treat hyperlipidemia less aggressively [37,38] and tend to avoid weight loss, at least in very old patients [39,40].

References

[1] Mungall M, Gaw A, Shephard J. Statin therapy in the elderly. Does it make good clinical and economic sense? Drugs Aging 2003;20(4):263–75.

[2] Grundy SM, Cleeman JI, Rifkind BM, et al. Cholesterol lowering in the elderly population. Coordinating Committee of the National Cholesterol Education Program. Arch Intern Med 1999;159(15):1670–8.

[3] National Lipid Education Council. Treating dyslipidemia in the elderly: are we doing enough? Lipid Management Newsletter 1999;4:1.

[4] Summary of the second report of the National Cholesterol Education Program (NCEP) Expert Panel on Detection, Evaluation, and Treatment of High Blood Cholesterol in Adults (Adult Treatment Panel II). JAMA 1993;269(23):3015–23.

[5] Ferrara A, Barrett-Connor C, Shan J. Total, LDL, and HDL cholesterol decrease with age in older men and women. The Rancho Bernardo Study 1984–1994. Circulation 1997;96(1):37–43.

[6] Kreisberg RA, Kasim S. Cholesterol metabolism and aging. Am J Med 1987;82(1B):54–60.

[7] Rader DJ, Hoeg JM, Brewer HB Jr. Quantitation of plasma apolipoproteins in the primary and secondary prevention of coronary artery disease. Ann Intern Med 1994;120(12):1012–25.

[8] Fredrickson DS. An international classification of hyperlipidemias and hyperlipoproteinemias. Ann Intern Med 1971;75(3):471–2.

[9] Rosenson RS, Shott S, Lu L, et al. Hypertriglyceridemia and other factors associated with plasma viscosity. Am J Med 2001;110(6):488–92.

[10] de Graaf J, Hak-Lemmers HL, Hectors MP, et al. Enhanced susceptibility to in vitro oxidation of the dense low density lipoprotein subfraction in healthy subjects. Arterioscler Thromb 1991;11(2):298–306.

[11] Wittrup HH, Tybjaerg-Hansen A, Nordestgaard BG. Lipoprotein lipase mutations, plasma lipids and lipoproteins, and risk of ischemic heart disease. A meta-analysis. Circulation 1999; 99(22):2901–7.

[12] Sprecher DL, Harris BV, Stein EA, et al. Higher triglycerides, lower high-density lipoprotein cholesterol, and higher systolic blood pressure in lipoprotein lipase-deficient heterozygotes. Circulation 1996;94(12):3239–45.

[13] Chait A, Brazg RL, Tribble DL, et al. Susceptibility of small, dense, low-density lipoproteins to oxidative modification in subjects with the atherogenic lipoprotein phenotype, pattern B. Am J Med 1993;94(4):350–6.

[14] Galeano NF, Al-Haideri M, Keyserman F, et al. Small dense low density lipoprotein has increased affinity for LDL receptor-independent cell surface binding sites: a potential mechanism for increased atherogenicity. J Lipid Res 1998;39(4):1263–73.

[15] Slyper AH. Low-density lipoprotein density and atherosclerosis. Unraveling the connection. JAMA 1994;272(4):305–8.

[16] Selby JV, Austin MA, Newman B, et al. LDL subclass phenotypes and the insulin resistance syndrome in women. Circulation 1993;88(2):381–7.

[17] Ross R. The pathogenesis of atherosclerosis: a perspective for the 1990s. Nature 1993; 362(6423):801–9.

[18] Braunstein JB, Cheng A, Cohn G, et al. Lipid disorders: justification of methods and goals of treatment. Chest 2001;120(3):979–88.

[19] Ansell BJ, Watson KE, Fogelman AM. An evidence-based assessment of the NCEP Adult Treatment Panel II Guidelines. JAMA 1999;282(21):2051–7.

[20] Grundy SM, Cleeman JI, Merz CN, et al. Implications of recent clinical trials for the National Cholesterol Education Program Adult Treatment Panel III Guidelines. Circulation 2004;110(2):227–39.

[21] Kagansky N, Levy S, Berner Y, et al. Cholesterol lowering in the older population: time for reassessment? QJM 2001;94(9):457–63.

[22] Kalantzi KJ, Milionis HJ, Mikhailidis DP, et al. Lipid lowering therapy in the elderly: is there a benefit? Curr Pharm Des 2006;12(30):3945–60.

[23] Lemaitre RN, Psaty BM, Heckbert SR, et al. Therapy with hydroxymethylglutaryl coenzyme a reductase inhibitors (statins) and associated risk of incident cardiovascular events in older adults: evidence from the Cardiovascular Health Study. Arch Intern Med 2002; 162(12):1395–400.

[24] Sever PS, Poulter NR, Dahlof B, et al. The ASCOT Investigators. The Anglo-Scandinavian Cardiac Outcomes Trial lipid lowering arm: extended observations 2 years after trial closure. Eur Heart J 2008;29:499–508.

[25] Aronow W. Treatment of older persons with hypercholesterolemia with and without cardiovascular disease. J Gerontol A Biol Sci Med Sci 2001;56A(3):M138–45.

[26] Dornbrook-Lavender KA, Roth MT, Pieper JA. Secondary prevention of coronary heart disease in the elderly. Ann Pharmacother 2003;37(12):1867–76.

[27] Lewis SJ, Moye LA, Sacks FM, et al. Effect of pravastatin on cardiovascular events in older patients with myocardial infarction and cholesterol levels in the average range. Results of the Cholesterol and Recurrent Events (CARE) trial. Ann Intern Med 1998;129(9):681–9.

[28] Ford I, Blauw GJ, Murphy MB, et al. A Prospective Study of Pravastatin in the Elderly at Risk (PROSPER). Curr Control Trials Cardiovasc Med 2002;3:1–8.

[29] LaRosa JC, He J, Vupputuri S. Effect of statins on risk of coronary disease. A meta-analysis of randomized controlled trials. JAMA 1999;282(24):2340–6.

[30] Roberts CG, Guallar E, Rodriguez A. Efficacy and safety of statin monotherapy in older adults: a meta-analysis. J Gerontol A Biol Sci Med Sci 2007;62(8):879–87.

[31] Deedwania P, Stone PH, Bairey Merz CN, et al. Effects of intensive versus moderate lipid-lowering therapy on myocardial ischemia in older patients with coronary heart disease. Circulation 2007;115(6):700–7.

[32] Lipka L, Sager P, Strony J, et al, Ezetimibe Study Group. Efficacy and safety of coadministration of ezetimibe and statins in elderly patients with primary hypercholesterolaemia. Drugs Aging 2004;21(15):1025–32.

[33] Feldman T, Davidson M, Shah A, et al. Comparison of the lipid-modifying efficacy and safety profiles of ezetimibe coadministered with simvastatin in older versus younger patients with primary hypercholesterolemia: a post Hoc analysis of subpopulations from three pooled clinical trials. Clin Ther 2006;28(6):849–59.

[34] Mendelson, Aronow WS. Underutilization of the measurement of serum low density lipoprotein cholesterol levels and of lipid lowering therapy in older patients who manifest arthersclerotic disease. J of Gerontology 2002;57:M398–400.

[35] Jackevicius CA, Mamdani M, Tu JV. Adherence with statin therapy in elderly patients with and without acute coronary syndromes. JAMA 2002;288(4):462–7.

[36] Benner JS, Glynn RJ, Mogun H, et al. Long-term persistence in use of statin therapy in elderly patients. JAMA 2002;288(4):455–61.

[37] Messinger-Rapport BJ, Morley JE, Thomas DR, et al. Intensive session: new approaches to medical issues in long-term care. J Am Med Dir Assoc 2007;8(7):421–33.

[38] Levenson SA, Morley JE. Evidence rocks in long-term care, but does it roll? J Am Med Dir Assoc 2007;8(8):493–501.

[39] Morley JE. Weight loss in the nursing home. J Am Med Dir Assoc 2007;8(4):201–4.

[40] Rolland Y, Kim MJ, Gammack JK, et al. Office management of weight loss in older persons. Am J Med 2006;119(12):1019–26.

ELSEVIER
SAUNDERS

CLINICS IN
GERIATRIC
MEDICINE

Clin Geriatr Med 24 (2008) 489–501

Hypertension and the Older Diabetic

Wilbert S. Aronow, MD

Divisions of Cardiology, Geriatrics, and Pulmonary/Critical Care,
Department of Medicine, Westchester Medical Center/New York Medical College,
Macy Pavilion, Room 138, Valhalla, NY 10595, USA

Hypertension (a systolic blood pressure of ≥140 mm Hg or a diastolic blood pressure of ≥90 mm Hg) is a common comorbidity in persons with diabetes mellitus, and its prevalence increases with advancing age [1,2]. Of 2,003 persons aged greater or equal to 60 years, mean age 80 years, living in the community and seen in an academic geriatrics practice, 325 (17%) had diabetes mellitus [1]. Of these 325 older diabetics, 252 (75%) had hypertension and 300 (90%) had hypertension or dyslipidemia [1].

Both diabetes mellitus and hypertension are independent risk factors for development in older persons of coronary artery disease [3–7], ischemic stroke [3–12], peripheral arterial disease [13–22], and of congestive heart failure [3,23,24]. Diabetics with hypertension have a higher prevalence and incidence of coronary artery disease, ischemic stroke, peripheral arterial disease, and of congestive heart failure than diabetics without hypertension. Table 1 shows in 335 older diabetics with a mean age of 80 years, the prevalence of clinical cardiovascular disease or target organ damage.

Table 2 shows that diabetes mellitus and hypertension are significant independent risk factors for new coronary events, for new ischemic stroke, for peropheral arterial disease, and for new congestive heart failure in elderly men and women. In 5,991 patients with a mean age of 73 years, hospitalized with congestive heart failure, 900 (16%) had diabetes mellitus, 41% of whom were women. Diabetes mellitus significantly increased mortality during 5-year to 8-year follow-up by 1.4 times in men with congestive heart failure and by 1.7 times in women with congestive heart failure [26].

Echocardiographic left ventricular hypertrophy increases, in elderly patients with hypertension, the incidence of new coronary events by 3.3 times in Blacks and by 2.7 times in Whites, the incidence of new ischemic stroke by 2.8 times in Blacks and by 3.3 times in Whites, and the incidence of new

E-mail address: wsaronow@aol.com

doi:10.1016/j.cger.2008.03.001

Table 1
Prevalence of clinical cardiovascular disease or target organ damage in 335 diabetics, mean age 80 years

Variable	%
Coronary artery disease	44
Stroke or transient cerebral ischemic attack	28
Peripheral arterial disease	26
Congestive heart failure	19
Abnormal left ventricular ejection fraction	40
Nephropathy	32
Echocardiographic left ventricular hypertrophy	71
Electrocardiographic left ventricular hypertrophy	16
Retinopathy	21
Neuropathy	14
Clinical cardiovascular disease or target organ damage	85

Adapted from Ness J, Nassimiha D, Feria MI, Aronow WS. Diabetes mellitus in older African Americans, Hispanics, and Whites in an academic hospital-based geriatrics practice. Coronary Artery Disease 1999;10:345.

congestive heart failure by 3.7 times in Blacks and by 3.5 times in Whites [4]. New coronary events, ischemic stroke, and congestive heart failure are especially increased in elderly diabetics with hyopertension and echocardiographic left ventricular hypertrophy.

Diabetics with a mean age of 63 years had a higher prevalence of unrecognized myocardial infarction [18%] than nondiabetics with a mean age of 63 years (7%), diagnosed by treadmill exercise sestamibi stress tests. Diabetics with a mean age of 63 years and with no history of angina pectoris also had a higher prevalence of silent myocardial ischemia (33%) than nondiabetics with a mean age of 63 years (18%), diagnosed by treadmill exercise sestamibi stress tests. In this study, hypertension was present in 201 out of 287 diabetics (70%) and in 159 out of 292 nondiabetics (54%) [27].

Table 2
Diabetes mellitus and hypertension are significant independent risk factors for coronary events, ischemic stroke, peripheral arterial disease, and congestive heart failure in elderly men and women

Variable	Relative risk	
	Diabetes metillus	Hypertension
Coronary events in 664 men, mean age 80 years [3]	1.9	2
Coronary events in 1,488 women, mean age 82 years [3]	1.8	1.6
Ischemic stroke in 664 men, mean age 80 years [8]	1.5	2.2
Ischemic stroke in 1,488 women, mean age 82 years [8]	1.5	2.4
Peripheral arterial disease in 437 men, mean age 80 years [13]	6.1	2.2
Peripheral arterial disease in 1,444 women, mean age 81 years [13]	3.6	2.8
Congestive heart failure in 2,737 men and women, mean age 81 years [24]	1.4	2.5

Diabetics with a mean age of 71 years and with microalbuminuria have more severe angiographic coronary artery disease than diabetics with a mean age of 71 years, without microalbuminuria [28]. Of 306 patients with a mean age of 57 years, with diabetes mellitus or hypertension, 111 (36%) had microalbuminuria. At 39-month follow-up, the incidence of new stroke or new myocardial infarction or death was significantly higher in patients with microalbuminuria (40%) than in patients without microalbuminuria (19%) [29].

In this study, 228 of 306 subjects (75%) were treated with angiotensin-converting enzyme (ACE) inhibitors or angiotensin receptor blockers (ARBs). Significant independent predictors of the time to development of either new stroke or new myocardial infarction or death were ACE inhibitors or ARBs (risk ratio = 0.21), echocardiographic left ventricular hypertrophy (risk ratio = 6.7), diabetes mellitus (risk ratio = 4.0), prior stroke (risk ratio = 4.0), and prior myocardial infarction (risk ratio = 3.7) [30].

Diabetic patients have a worse prognosis than nondiabetic patients after percutaneous coronary revascularization [31–34]. However, in a study of 216 diabetics with a mean age of 66 years, and 552 nondiabetics with a mean age of 66 years, undergoing percutaneous coronary revascularization in which 99% of the subjects were treated with aspirin, 98% with clopidogrel, 85% with beta-blockers, and 96% with lipid lowering drugs, the incidence of in-hospitalization mortality or nonfatal myocardial infarction or nonfatal stroke was only 1.4% in diabetics versus 1.1% in nondiabetics [25].

Diabetic patients also have a worse prognosis than nondiabetics following surgical coronary revascularization [35]. In the Bypass Angioplasty Revascularization Investigation (BARI), the overall 5-year survival rate was 89% for the coronary artery bypass graft group versus 86% for the percutaneous coronary revascularization group (*P* not significant) [36]. However, in the subgroup of patients with diabetes mellitus, the 5-year survival was significantly improved in the coronary artery bypass group (76%) versus the percutaneous coronary revascularization group (56%) [36].

Treatment of elderly diabetics with hypertension

Because elderly diabetics with hypertension are at a very high risk for developing fatal and nonfatal coronary heart disease, fatal stroke and nonfatal stroke or transient cerebral ischemic attack, peripheral arterial disease, congestive heart failure, nephropathy, left ventricular hypertrophy, and other target organ damage, these patients should have intensive treatment of modifiable risk factors. Cigarette smoking must be stopped, with a smoking cessation program instituted if necessary (Box 1) [37].

Elderly diabetics should have their hemoglobin A_{1c} level reduced to less than 7% [37,38]. Diabetics have a significant increasing trend of hemoglobin

---

Box 1. Treatment of elderly diabetics with hypertension

Cigarette smoking must be stopped and a smoking cessation
    program instituted if necessary.

Obesity must be treated by diet and aerobic exercise, and the
    body mass index reduced to 18.5 kg/m^2–24.9 kg/m^2.

Reduce hemoglobin A$_{1c}$ level to less than 7%.

Treat dyslipidemia with the serum low-density
    lipoprotein cholesterol reduced to less than 70 mg/dL
    in very high-risk persons.

Serum triglycerides should be less than 150 mg/dL
    and serum high-density lipoprotein cholesterol
    should be greater than 40 mg/dL.

Treat with aspirin.

Treat with angiotensin-converting enzyme inhibitors and
    beta-blockers if there is prior myocardial infarction or abnormal
    left ventricular ejection fraction.

Reduce blood pressure to less than 130/80 mm Hg.

Choice of initial antihypertensive drug will depend on associated
    comorbidities.

Angiotensin-converting enzyme inhibitors or angiotensin
    receptor blockers should be used to treat hypertension,
    especially if nephropathy is present; multiple antihypertensive
    drugs are often needed to control blood pressure.

A$_{1c}$ levels over the increasing number of vessels with coronary artery disease
[39]. The higher the hemoglobin A$_{1c}$ level in diabetics with a mean age of
70 years with peripheral arterial disease, the more severe the peripheral
arterial disease as measured by the ankle-brachial index (ABI). In the study
by Aronow and colleagues [40], the prevalence of hypertension was 75% in
135 diabetics with an ABI of 0.60 to 0.89, and 78% in 89 diabetics with an
ABI of less than 0.60.

Elderly diabetics are more often obese and have higher serum low-density
lipoprotein (LDL) cholesterol and triglycerides levels and lower serum high-
density lipoprotein (HDL) cholesterol levels than do nondiabetics. These
risk factors contribute to the higher incidence of cardiovascular morbidity
and mortality in diabetics than in nondiabetics. Regular aerobic exercise
should be added to diet in treating obesity. The body mass index should
be reduced to a range of 18.5 kg/m^2 to 24.9 kg/m^2 (see Box 1) [37].

Dyslipidemia must be treated in elderly diabetics with hypertension
[41–45]. The Heart Protection Study showed that in 20,536 persons, those
at high risk for cardiovascular events should be treated with statins, regardless of the initial levels of serum lipids, age, or gender [41].

In the Collaborative Atorvastatin Diabetes Study, 2,838 subjects with a mean age of 62 years with diabetes mellitus, no cardiovascular disease, and a serum LDL cholesterol less than 160 mg/dL were randomized to atorvastatin 10-mg daily or placebo [43]. At the 3.9-year median follow-up, compared with placebo, atorvastatin significantly reduced time to first occurrence of acute coronary events, coronary revascuarization, or stroke by 37%, acute coronary events by 36%, and stroke by 48% [43].

In an observational prospective study of 529 subjects with a mean age of 79 years and with prior myocardial infarction, diabetes mellitus, and a serum LDL cholesterol of 125 mg/dL or higher, 53% of subjects were treated with statins. At the 29-month follow-up, compared with no treatment with statins, use of statins significantly decreased coronary heart death or nonfatal myocardial infarction by 37% and stroke by 47%. In this study, 83% of diabetics treated with statins had hypertension [44].

Elderly diabetics with hypertension should have their serum LDL cholesterol level reduced to less than 70 mg/dL. When a high-risk person has hypertriglyceridemia or low serum HDL cholesterol, consideration can be given to combining a fibrate or nicotinic acid with an LDL cholesterol-lowering drug (see Box 1) [45]. The American Diabetes Association recommends serum triglycerides of less than 150 mg/dL and a serum HDL cholesterol of greater than 40 mg/dL in diabetics [38].

Diabetics with macrovascular disease or with one or more cardiovascular risk factors, such as hypertension, should be treated with aspirin 75 mg to 325 mg daily [37,38]. At the 3.8-year follow-up in the Hypertension Optimal Treatment trial of 18,790 patients with a mean age of 62 years, 1,501 diabetics had a significant 51% reduction in major cardiovascular events if they were randomized to a target group of diastolic blood pressure of less than or equal to 80 mm Hg, compared with a target group of a diastolic blood of less than or equal to 90 mm Hg (Box 2) [46]. In this study, subjects randomized to aspirin had a significant reduction in major cardiovascular events of 15% and in myocardial infarction of 36%, with no effect on stroke [46].

Elderly diabetics with hypertension and prior myocardial infarction should be treated with ACE inhibitors and beta-blockers (see Box 1) [37,54–60]. The Joint National Committee 7 on Detection, Evaluation, and Treatment of High Blood Pressure also recommends use of aldosterone antagonists in the treatment of hypertension after myocardial infarction in the absence of hyperkalemia or significant renal dysfunction [54,61].

An observational prospective study was performed in 477 subjects with a mean age of 79 years, with prior myocardial infarction and a mean left ventricular ejection fraction of 31% [56]. At the 34-month follow-up, subjects treated with beta-blockers without ACE inhibitors had a 25% significant reduction in new coronary events and a 41% significant reduction in congestive heart failure. At the 34-month follow-up, subjects treated with ACE inhibitors had a significant 17% reduction in new coronary events and

Box 2. Studies of antihypertensive drugs in diabetics

Hypertension Optimal Treatment Trial [46]
At 3 to 8 year follow-up of 1,501 hypertensive diabetics
    randomized to antihypertensive therapy, major cardiovascular
    events were reduced 51% if they were randomized to a target
    group of a diastolic blood pressure of less than or equal to
    80 mm Hg, compared with a target group of a diastolic
    blood pressure of less than or equal to 90 mm Hg

United Kingdom Prospective Diabetes Study [47]
At the 8.4-year follow-up of 1,148 hypertensive diabetics,
    each 10-mm Hg reduction in systolic blood pressure was
    associated with reductions in risk of 12% for any
    complication related to diabetes, of 15% for deaths
    related to diabetes, of 11% for myocardial infarction,
    and of 13% for microvascular complications

Heart Outcomes Prevention Evaluation Study [48]
At the 4.5-year follow-up of 3,577 diabetics randomized
    to ramipril or placebo, ramipril reduced all-cause
    mortality by 24% and myocardial infarction, stroke,
    or cardiovascular death by 25%

Appropriate Blood Pressure Control in Diabetes Trial [49]
At the 5-year follow-up of 53 hypertensive diabetics with
    peripheral arterial disease, the incidence of myocardial
    infarction, stroke, or cardiovascular death was 14% in subjects
    in whom the blood pressure was reduced to 128/75 mm Hg,
    compared with 39% in subjects in whom the blood pressure
    was reduced to 137/81 mm Hg

Appropriate Blood Pressure Control in Diabetes Trial [50]
At the 5-year follow-up of 470 hypertensive diabetics, patients
    randomized to nisoldipine had a five times increase in fatal
    and nonfatal myocardial infarction, compared with patients
    randomized to enalapril

*Fosinopril versus Amlodipine Cardiovascular Events
Randomized Trial [51]*
At the 3.5-year follow-up of 380 hypertensive diabetics,
    compared with those randomized to amlodipine, those
    randomized to fosinopril had a 51% reduction in combined
    incidence of fatal and nonfatal stroke, fatal and nonfatal
    myocardial infarction, and hospitalization for angina pectoris

---

Antihypertensive and Lipid-Lowering Treatment to Prevent Heart Attack Trial [52]

At the 3.3-year follow-up of 14,000 hypertensive diabetics, compared with chlorthalidone, doxazosin increased combined cardiovascular events by 25%, stroke by 19%, congestive heart failure by 204%, and angina pectoris by 16%

Antihypertensive and Lipid-Lowering Treatment to Prevent Heart Attack Trial [53]

At the 4.9-year follow-up of 14,000 hypertensive diabetics, compared with chlorthalidone, the primary outcome of fatal coronary heart disease or nonfatal myocardial infarction was similar in patients randomized to lisinopril or amlodipine

---

a significant 32% reduction in congestive heart failure. At the 41-month follow-up, subjects treated with both beta-blockers and ACE inhibitors had a significant 37% reduction in new coronary events and a significant 60% reduction in congestive heart failure [56].

In an observational prospective study of 1,212 older men and women with a mean age of 80 years, with prior myocardial infarction and hypertension treated with beta-blockers, ACE inhibitors, diuretics, calcium channel blockers, or alpha-blockers, at 40-month follow-up the incidence of new coronary events in persons treated with one antihypertensive drug was lowest in persons treated with beta-blockers or ACE inhibitors [58]. In older persons treated with two antihypertensive drugs, the incidence of new coronary events was lowest in persons treated with beta-blockers plus ACE inhibitors [57].

In 613 patients with a mean age of 79 years, with diabetes mellitus and prior myocardial infarction, 76% had hypertension. Patients treated with beta-blockers (53% of group without contraindications) had a significant 27% independent reduction in new coronary events at the 33-month follow-up [57].

Antihypertensive studies in diabetics

Patients with diabetes mellitus or with chronic renal insufficiency, which may be present in diabetics, should have their blood pressure reduced to less than 130/80 mm Hg [37,38,54,62]. Often, multiple antihypertensive drugs will be required to meet this goal [38,54,63–65].

In the United Kingdom Prospective Diabetes Study, 1,148 diabetics with hypertension and a mean age 56 years, were randomized to treatment with atenolol or captopril (see Box 2) [47]. At the 8.4-year follow-up, each 10-mm Hg reduction in systolic blood pressure was associated with significant reductions in risk of 12% for any complication related to diabetes, of 15% for deaths related to diabetes, of 11% for myocardial infarction, and of 13% for microvascular complications. The lowest risk occurred in diabetics with a systolic blood pressure of less than 120 mm Hg. Captopril and atenolol were equally effective in reducing complications.

In the Heart Outcomes Prevention Evaluation Study, 3,577 diabetics aged 55 years and older with a mean age of 66 years, were randomized to ramipril or placebo (see Box 2) [48]. At the 4.5-year follow-up, compared with placebo, ramipril significantly reduced the primary outcome of myocardial infarction, stroke, or cardiovascular death by 25%, all-cause mortality by 24%, myocardial infarction by 22%, stroke by 33%, cardiovascular death by 37%, revascularization by 17%, and overt nephropathy by 24%.

At the 5-year follow-up of 53 hypertensive diabetics with peripheral arterial disease and a mean age of 60 years in the Appropriate Blood Pressure Control in Diabetes Trial (see Box 2), the incidence of myocardial infarction, stroke, or cardiovascular death was significantly less for those in whom the blood pressure was reduced to 128/75 mm Hg (14%) than in patients in whom the blood pressure was reduced to 137/81 mm Hg (39%) [49]. In this study, at the 5-year follow-up of 470 hypertensive diabetics with a mean age of 60 years, subjects randomized to nisoldipine had a five times significantly increased incidence of fatal and nonfatal myocardial infarction, compared with patients randomized to enalapril [50].

At 3.5-year follow-up of 380 diabetics with hypertension and a mean age of 63 years, compared with subjects randomized to amlodipine, subjects randomized to fosinopril had a 51% significant reduction in the combined incidence of fatal and nonfatal stroke, fatal and nonfatal myocardial infarction, and hospitalization for angina pectoris [51].

In the Antihypertensive and Lipid-Lowering Treatment to Prevent Heart Attack Trial (see Box 2), 14,000 diabetics with a mean age of 67 years, with hypertension were randomized to chlorthalidone, doxazosin, lisinopril, or amlodipine [52,53]. At the 3.3-year follow-up, compared with chlorthalidone, doxazosin significantly increased combined cardiovascular events by 25%, stroke by 19%, congestive heart failure by 204%, and angina pectoris by 16%, and was discontinued from the study [52]. At the 4.9-year follow-up, compared with chlorthalidone, the primary outcome of fatal coronary heart disease or nonfatal myocardial infartion was similar in subjects randomized to lisinopril or to amlodipine [53].

On the basis of the available data, the reduction of macrovascular and microvascular complications in elderly diabetics with hypertension depends more on reducing the blood pressure to less than 130/80 mm Hg than on the type of antihypertensive drugs used. The choice of antihypertensive drugs initially used depends on the associated comorbidities [38,54,66].

For example, elderly hypertensive diabetics with prior myocardial infarction or abnormal left ventricular ejection fraction should be treated with ACE inhibitors and beta-blockers [37,54–60]. Patients with congestive heart failure should be treated with diuretics, ACE inhibitors, and beta-blockers [67,68]. Elderly hypertensive diabetics with nephropathy should be treated initially with ACE inhibitors or ARBs [54,69–72]. Multiple antihypertensive drugs will often need to be used to reduce the blood pressure to less than 130/80 mm Hg.

References

[1] Ness J, Nassimiha D, Feria MI, et al. Diabetes mellitus in older African-Americans, Hispanics, and Whites in an academic hospital-based geriatrics practice. Coron Artery Dis 1999;10:343–6.

[2] Oldridge NB, Stump TE, Nothwehr FK, et al. Prevalence and outcomes of comorbid metabolic and cardiovascular conditions in middle-and older-age adults. J Clin Epidemiol 2001;54:928–34.

[3] Aronow WS, Ahn C. Risk factors for new coronary events in a large cohort of very elderly patients with and without coronary artery disease. Am J Cardiol 1996;77:864–6.

[4] Aronow WS, Ahn C, Kronzon I, et al. Congestive heart failure, coronary events and athero-thrombotic brain infarction in elderly Blacks and Whites with systemic hypertension and with and without echocardiographic and electrocardiographic evidence of left ventricular hypertrophy. Am J Cardiol 1991;67:295–9.

[5] Vokonas PS, Kannel WB. Epidemiology of coronary heart disease in the elderly. In: Aronow WS, Fleg JL, editors. Cardiovascular disease in the elderly. 3rd edition. Revised and expanded. New York: Marcel Dekker, Inc.; 2004. p. 189–214.

[6] Haffner SM, Lehto S, Ronnemaa T, et al. Mortality from coronary heart disease in subjects with type 2 diabetes and in nondiabetic subjects with and without prior myocardial infarction. N Engl J Med 1998;339:229–34.

[7] Aronow WS, Ahn C. Elderly diabetics with peripheral arterial disease and no coronary artery disease have a higher incidence of new coronary events than elderly nondiabetics with peripheral arterial disease and prior myocardial infarction treated with statins and with no lipid-lowering drug. J Gerontol A Biol Sci Med Sci 2003;58A:M573–5.

[8] Aronow WS, Ahn C, Gutstein H. Risk factors for new atherothrombotic brain infarction in 664 older men and 1,488 older women. Am J Cardiol 1996;77:1381–3.

[9] Garland C, Barrett-Connor E, Suarez L, et al. Isolated systolic hypertension and mortality after age 60 years. Am J Epidemiol 1983;118:365–76.

[10] SHEP Cooperative Research Group: prevention of stroke by antihypertensive drug treatment in older persons with isolated systolic hypertension: final results of the systolic hypertension in the elderly program (SHEP). JAMA 1991;265:3255–64.

[11] Barrett-Connor E, Khaw KT. Diabetes mellitus: an independent risk factor for stroke. Am J Epidemiol 1988;128:116–23.

[12] Weinberger J. Cerebrovascular disease in the elderly patient. In: Aronow WS, Fleg JL, editors. Cardiovascular disease in the elderly. 3rd edition. Revised and expanded. New York: Marcel Dekker, Inc.,; 2004. p. 625–51.

[13] Ness J, Aronow WS, Ahn C. Risk factors for peripheral arterial disease in an academic hospital-based geriatrics practice. J Am Geriatr Soc 2000;48:312–4.

[14] Hughson WG, Mann JI, Garrod A. Intermittent claudication: prevalence and risk factors. Br Med J 1978;1:1379–81.

[15] Schroll M, Munck O. Estimation of peripheral arteriosclerotic disease by ankle blood pressure measurements in a population of 60 year old men and women. J Chronic Dis 1981;34:261–9.

[16] Beach KW, Brunzell JD, Strandness DE Jr. Prevalence of severe arteriosclerosis obliterans in patients with diabetes mellitus: relation to smoking and form of therapy. Arteriosclerosis 1982;2:275–80.

[17] Reunanen A, Takkunen H, Aromaa A. Prevalence of intermittent claudication and its effect on mortality. Acta Med Scand 1982;211:249–56.

[18] Pomrehn P, Duncan B, Weissfeld L, et al. The association of dyslipoproteinemia with symptoms and signs of peripheral arterial disease: the Lipid Research Clinics Program prevalence study. Circulation 1986;73(Suppl I):I-100–7.

[19] Stokes J III, Kannel WB, Wolf PA, et al. The relative importance of selected risk factors for various manifestations of cardiovascular disease among men and women from 35 to 64 years old: 30 years of follow-up in the Framingham study. Circulation 1987;75(Suppl V):V65–73.

[20] Aronow WS, Sales FF, Etienne F, et al. Prevalence of peripheral arterial disease and its correlation with risk factors for peripheral arterial disease in elderly patients in a long-term health care facility. Am J Cardiol 1988;62:644–6.

[21] Beach KW, Brunzell JD, Conquest LL, et al. The correlation of arteriosclerosis obliterans with lipoproteins in insulin-dependent and non-insulin-dependent diabetes. Diabetes 1979; 28:836–40.

[22] Ness J, Aronow WS, Newkirk E, et al. Prevalence of asymptomatic peripheral arterial disease, modifiable risk factors, and appropriate use of drugs in the treatment of peripheral arterial disease in older persons seen in a university general medicine clinic. J Gerontol A Biol Sci Med Sci 2005;60A:255–7.

[23] Kannel WB, Hjortland M, Castelli WP. Role of diabetes in congestive heart failure: the Framingham study. Am J Cardiol 1974;34:29–34.

[24] Aronow WS, Ahn C. Incidence of heart failure in 2,737 older persons with and without diabetes mellitus. Chest 1999;115:867–8.

[25] Gustafsson I, Brendorp B, Seibaek M, et al. Influence of diabetes and diabetes-gender interaction on the risk of death in patients hospitalized with congestive heart failure. J Am Coll Cardiol 2004;43:771–7.

[26] Gamble SM, Saulle LN, Aronow WS, et al. Incidence of in-hospital mortality or nonfatal myocardial infarction or nonfatal stroke in 216 diabetics and 552 nondiabetics undergoing percutaneous coronary intervention with stenting. Am J Therap 2007;14:435–7.

[27] DeLuca AJ, Kaplan S, Aronow WS, et al. Comparison of prevalence of unrecognized myocardial infarction and of silent myocardial ischemia detected by a treadmill exercise sestamibi stress test in patients with versus without diabetes mellitus. Am J Cardiol 2006;98:1045–6.

[28] Sukhija R, Aronow WS, Kakar P, et al. Relation of microalbuminuria and coronary artery disease in patients with and without diabetes mellitus. Am J Cardiol 2006;98:279–81.

[29] Ravipati G, Aronow WS, Ahn C, et al. Incidence of new stroke or new myocardial infarction or death at 39-month follow-up in patients with diabetes mellitus or systemic hypertension with and without microalbuminuria. Cardiology 2008;109:62–5.

[30] Ravipati G, Aronow WS, Ahn C, et al. Incidence of new stroke or new myocardial infarction or death at 39-month follow-up in patients with diabetes mellitus, hypertension, or both treated with and without angiotensin-converting enzyme inhibitors or angiotensin receptor blockers. Am J Therap, in press.

[31] Elezi S, Kastrati A, Pache J, et al. Diabetes mellitus and the clinical and angiographic outcome after coronary stent placement. J Am Coll Cardiol 1998;32:1866–73.

[32] Kip KE, Faxon DP, Detre KM, et al. Coronary angioplasty in diabetic patients: the National Heart, Lung, And Blood Institute Percutaneous Transluminal Coronary Angioplasty Registry. Circulation 1996;94:1818–25.

[33] Levine GN, Jacobs AK, Keeler GP, et al. Impact of diabetes mellitus on percutaneous revascularization (CAVEAT-1). Am J Cardiol 1997;79:748–55.

[34] Abizaid A, Kornowski R, Mintz GS, et al. The influence of diabetes mellitus on acute and late clinical outcomes following coronary stent implantation. J Am Coll Cardiol 1998;32: 584–9.

[35] Detre KM, Lombardero MS, Brooks MM, et al. The effect of previous coronary -artery bypass surgery on the prognosis of patients with diabetes who have acute myocardial infarction. N Engl J Med 2000;342:989–97.

[36] Frye FL, Alderman E, Bourassa M, et al. Influence of diabetes on 5-year mortality and morbidity in a randomized trial comparing CABG and PTCA in patients with multivessel disease: the Bypass Angioplasty Revascularization Investigation (BARI). Circulation 1997;96:1761–9.

[37] Smith SC Jr, Allen J, Blair SN, et al. ACC/AHA guidelines for secondary prevention for patients with coronary and other atherosclerotic vascular disease: 2006 update: endorsed by the National Heart, Lung, and Blood Institute. Circulation 2006;113:2363–72.

[38] American Diabetes Association. Standards of medical care for patients with diabetes mellitus. Diabetes Care 2003;26(Suppl 1):S33–50.

[39] Ravipati G, Aronow WS, Ahn C, et al. Association of hemoglobin A_{1c} level with the severity of coronary artery disease in patients with diabetes mellitus. Am J Cardiol 2006;97:968–9.

[40] Aronow WS, Ahn C, Weiss MB, et al Relation of hemoglobin A1c levels to severity of peripheral arterial disease in patients with diabetes mellitus. Am J Cardiol 2007;99:1468–9.

[41] Heart Protection Study Collaborative Group. MRC/BHF heart protection study of cholesterol lowering with simvastatin in 20,536 high-risk individuals: a randomised placebo-controlled trial. Lancet 2002;360:7–22.

[42] Sever PS, Dahlof B, Poulter NR, et al. Prevention of coronary and stroke events with atorvastatin in hypertensive patients who have average or lower-than-average cholesterol concentrations, in the Anglo-Scandinavian Cardiac Outcomes Trial—lipid lowering arm (ASCOT-LLA): a multicentre randomised controlled trial. Lancet 2003;361:1149–58.

[43] Calhoun HM, Betteridge DJ, Durrington PN, et al. Primary prevention of cardiovascular disease with atorvastatin in type 2 diabetes mellitus in the Collaborative Atorvastatin Diabetes Study (CARDS): multicentre randomized placebo-controlled trial. Lancet 2004; 364:685–96.

[44] Aronow WS, Ahn C, Gutstein H. Reduction of new coronary events and of new atherothrombotic brain infarction in older persons with diabetes mellitus, prior myocardial infarction, and serum low-density lipoprotein cholesterol ≥ 125 mg/dL treated with statins. J Gerontol A Biol Sci Med Sci 2002;57A:M747–50.

[45] Grundy SM, Cleeman JI, Merz CN, et al. Implications of recent clinical trials for the National Cholesterol Education Program Adult Treatment Panel III guidelines. Circulation 2004;110:227–39.

[46] Hansson L, Zanchetti A, Carruthers SG, et al. Effects of intensive blood-pressure lowering and low-dose aspirin in patients with hypertension: principal result of the hypertension optimal treatment (HOT) randomised trial. Lancet 1998;351:1755–62.

[47] Adler AI, Stratton IM, Neil HAW, et al. Association of systolic blood pressure with macrovascular and microvascular complications of type 2 diabetes (UKPDS 36): prospective observational study. Br Med J 2000;321:412–9.

[48] Heart Outcomes Prevention Evaluation (HOPE) Study Investigators. Effects of ramipril on cardiovascular and microvascular outcomes in people with diabetes mellitus: results of the HOPE study and MICRO-HOPE substudy. Lancet 2000;355:253–9.

[49] Mehler PS, Coll JR, Estacio R, et al. Intensive blood pressure control reduces the risk of cardiovascular events in patients with peripheral arterial disease and type 2 diabetes. Circulation 2003;107:753–6.

[50] Estacio RO, Jeffers BW, Hiatt WR, et al. The effect of nisoldipine as compared with enalapril on cardiovascular outcomes in patients with non-insulin-dependent diabetes and hypertension. N Engl J Med 1998;338:645–52.

[51] Tatti P, Pahor M, Byington RP, et al. Outcome results of the fosinopril versus amlodipine cardiovascular events randomized trial (FACET) in patients with hypertenson and NIDDM. Diabetes Care 1998;21:597–603.

[52] ALLHAT Officers and Coordinators for the ALLHAT Collaborative Research Group. Major cardiovascular events in hypertensive patients randomized to doxazosin vs chlorthalidone. The antihypertensive and lipid-lowering treatment to prevent heart attack trial (ALLHAT). JAMA 2000;283:1967–75.

[53] ALLHAT Officers and Coordinators for the ALLHAT Collaborative Research Group. Major outcomes in high-risk hypertensive patients randomized to angiotensin-converting enzyme inhibitor or calcium channel blocker vs diuretic. The antihypertensive and lipid-lowering treatment to prevent heart attack trial (ALLHAT). JAMA 2002;288:2981–97.

[54] Chobanian AV, Bakris GL, Black HR, et al. The seventh report of the Joint National Committee on Prevention, Detection, Evaluation, and Treatment of High Blood Pressure. The JNC 7 report. JAMA 2003;289:2560–72.

[55] The Heart Outcomes Prevention Evaluation Study Investigators. Effects of an angiotensin-converting-enzyme inhibitor, ramipril on cardiovascular events in high-risk patients. N Engl J Med 2000;342:145–53.

[56] Aronow WS, Ahn C, Kronzon I. Effect of beta blockers alone, of angiotensin-converting enzyme inhibitors alone, and of beta blockers plus angiotensin-converting enzyme inhibitors on new coronary events and on congestive heart failure in older persons with healed myocardial infarcts and asymptomatic left ventricular systolic dysfunction. Am J Cardiol 2001;88:1298–300.

[57] Aronow WS, Ahn C. Effect of beta blockers on incidence of new coronary events in older persons with prior myocardial infarction and diabetes mellitus. Am J Cardiol 2001;87:780–1.

[58] Aronow WS, Ahn C. Incidence of new coronary events in older persons with prior myocardial infarction and systemic hypertension treated with beta blockers, angiotensin-converting enzyme inhibitors, diuretics, calcium antagonists, and alpha blockers. Am J Cardiol 2002;89:1207–9.

[59] Pfeffer MA, Braunwald E, Moye LA, et al. Effect of captopril on mortality and morbidity in patients with left ventricular dysfunction after myocardial infarction. Results of the survival and ventricular enlargement trial. N Engl J Med 1992;327:669–77.

[60] The European trial on reduction of cardiac events with perindopril in stable coronary artery disease investigators. Efficacy of perindopril in reduction of cardiovascular events among patients with stable coronary artery disease: randomised, double-blind, placebo-controlled, multicentre trial (the EUROPA study). Lancet 2003;362:782–8.

[61] Pitt B, Remme W, Zannad F, et al. Eplerenone, a selective aldosterone blocker, in patients with left ventricular dysfunction after myocardial infarction. N Engl J Med 2003;348:1309–21.

[62] Bakris GL, Williams M, Dworkin L. For National Kidney Foundation Hypertension and Diabetes Executive Committees Working Group. Preserving renal function in adults with hypertension and diabetes. Am J Kidney Dis 2000;36:646–61.

[63] American Diabetes Association. Treatment of hypertension of adults with diabetes. Diabetes Care 2003;26(Suppl 1):580–2.

[64] National Kidney Foundation Guideline. K/DOQI clinical practice guidelines for chronic kidney disease: Kidney disease outcome quality initiative. Am J Kidney Dis 2002;39(Suppl 2):S1–246.

[65] Gandelman G, Aronow WS, Varma R. Prevalence of adequate blood pressure control in self-pay or Medicare patients versus Medicaid or private insurance patients with systemic hypertension followed in a university cardiology or general medicine clinic. Am J Cardiol 2004;94:815–6.

[66] Aronow WS. Drug therapy of older persons with hypertension. J Am Med Dir Assoc 2006;7:193–6.

[67] Hunt SA, Abraham WT, Feldman AM, et al. ACC/AHA 2005 guideline update for the diagnosis and management of chronic heart failure in the adult-summary article. A report of the American College of Cardiology/American Heart Association Task Force on practice guidelines (writing committee to update the 2001 guidelines for the evaluation and management of heart failure). Developed in collaboration with the American College of Chest Physicians and the International Society for Heart and Lung Transplantation. Endorsed by the Heart Rhythm Society. J Am Coll Cardiol 2005;46:1116–43.

[68] Aronow WS. Epidemiology, pathophysiology, prognosis, and treatment of systolic and diastolic heart failure. Cardiol Rev 2006;14:108–24.

[69] Agodoa LY, Appel L, Bakris GL, et al. Effect of ramipril versus amlodipine on renal outcomes in hypertensive nephrosclerosis. A randomized controlled trial. JAMA 2001; 285:2719–28.

[70] Brenner BM, Cooper ME, de Zeeuw D, et al. Effects of losartan on renal and cardiovascular outcomes in patients with type 2 diabetes and nephropathy. N Engl J Med 2001;345:861–9.

[71] Beri T, Hunsicker LG, Lewis JB, et al. Cardiovascular outcomes in the Irbesartan diabetic nephropathy trial of patients with type 2 diabetes and overt nephropathy. Ann Intern Med 2003;138:542–9.

[72] Strippoli GF, Craig MC, Schena FP, et al. Role of blood pressure targets and specific anti-hypertensive agents used to prevent diabetic nephropathy and delay its progression. J Am Soc Nephrol 2006;17(Suppl 2):S153–5.

ELSEVIER
SAUNDERS

CLINICS IN
GERIATRIC
MEDICINE

Clin Geriatr Med 24 (2008) 503–513

Nutrition and the Older Diabetic

Neelavathi Senkottaiyan, MD

*Division of Endocrinology, Saint Louis University Medical Center,
1402 South Grand Boulevard, Donco Building, 2nd Floor, St. Louis, MO 63104, USA*

Diabetes mellitus is among the most common and complex chronic diseases that affect approximately 20 million individuals in the United States. An additional 26% of the population has impaired fasting glucose, making diabetes an epidemic [1,2].

Results from the Diabetes Control and Complications Trial and United Kingdom Prospective Diabetes Study convincingly show the importance of glycemic control in preventing the microvascular complications of diabetes [3,4]. In both trials, medical nutrition therapy (MNT) was important in achieving treatment goals.

MNT in diabetes addresses not only glycemic control but also other aspects of metabolic status, including hypertension and dyslipidemia, which are major risk factors for cardiovascular disease. MNT is an integral component of diabetes management, which includes the process and system through which nutritional care and specific life style recommendations are provided to diabetic individuals. Cultural and ethnic preferences are taken into account and patients are involved in the decision-making process.

Before 1994, the American Diabetes Association attempted to define an ideal and standard nutrition prescription for everyone who had diabetes [5]. The 1994 nutrition recommendation shifted to emphasize the effects of nutritional therapy on metabolic control [6].

The goal of MNT is to assist and facilitate individual lifestyle and behavior changes that will lead to improved metabolic control. The recommendations are based on promoting optimal nutrition through healthy food choices and an active lifestyle. Outcome studies have shown that MNT provided by registered dietitian results in a 1.0% decrease in HbA1c in patients who have newly diagnosed type 1 diabetes, a 2.0% decrease in patients who have newly diagnosed type 2 diabetes, and a 1.0% decrease in patients who had type 2 diabetes for an average of 4 years.

E-mail address: nsenkott@slu.edu

0749-0690/08/$ - see front matter © 2008 Elsevier Inc. All rights reserved.
doi:10.1016/j.cger.2008.03.010   *geriatric.theclinics.com*

Biologic changes of aging

Aging is associated with many biologic changes that may predispose older adults to nutritional deficiencies. These changes include alterations in taste, smell, mastication, salivary flow, gastric acidity, hepatic, and renal function [7]. In addition, difficulty in preparing food, polypharmacy, and alcoholism are common problems that may interfere with adequate nutrition. Because of these concerns, any nutritional intervention must start with a thorough assessment of clinical, nutritional history, and psychosocial and environmental evaluation.

Limited research exists on the changes in nutritional needs with aging, and virtually none is available on aging patients who have diabetes. Therefore, nutritional recommendations for older patients who have diabetes must be extrapolated from the general population.

The most reliable indicator of poor nutritional status in older individuals is change in body weight. Involuntary loss of more than 10 lb or 5% of body weight in less than 6 months should be evaluated to determine nutritional status [8,9].

Because of the changes in body composition caused by loss of lean body mass and altered exercise patterns, the energy requirements of older adults are 20% to 30% lower than in younger adults [10]. Studies have shown that the resting metabolic rate is lower in elderly patients even after adjusting for lean body mass [11]. Nevertheless, the need for weight loss in overweight older adults should be carefully evaluated.

Older diabetic patients, especially those in a nursing home, tend to be under- rather than overweight [12,13]. Low body weight has been associated with greater morbidity and mortality in this age group [14], and weight loss in older diabetics was associated with increased mortality [15].

Aging does not seem to alter the synthesis or breakdown rate of protein when adjusted for fat free mass [16]. Older subjects do not show impairment in energy conservation or disposition during experimental conditions of under- or overfeeding [17].

In long-term care settings, malnutrition and dehydration may develop because of lack of food choices, poor food quality, and unnecessary dietary restrictions [17–20]. Specialized diabetic diets do not seem superior to standard unrestricted diets in these settings [21–23]. Therefore, the recommendation is that residents be served the regular menu with consistent amounts of carbohydrates for meals and snacks. Changing medication to control blood glucose is often preferable to implementing food restrictions.

Macronutrients

Carbohydrates

Studies in healthy subjects and those at risk for type 2 diabetes support the importance of a diet containing carbohydrates from whole grains, fruits, vegetables, and low-fat milk [24,25]. Regarding glycemic effect of carbohydrates, the total amount of carbohydrates in meals or snacks is more important than its source. Although foods with low glycemic index may reduce postprandial blood glucose excursions, little evidence supports the general use of a low glycemic diet.

Consumption of fiber should be encouraged. Although large amounts (50 g/d) of fiber may have beneficial effects on glycemia, insulinemia, and lipemia, whether high fiber intake can be maintained long-term is unknown because of gastrointestinal side effects [26].

Nutritive sweeteners

Sucrose and sucrose-containing foods need not be restricted in patients who have diabetes, because clinical studies show that dietary sucrose does not increase glycemia more than isocaloric amounts of starch [27]. Fructose accounts for 9% of average energy intake in the United States; 33% of dietary fructose comes from fruits and vegetables, and 67% comes from added fructose in food and beverages. In several studies, fructose decreased postprandial blood glucose when it replaced sucrose or starch as a carbohydrate source.

Nonnutritive sweeteners

Nonnutritive sweeteners are safe for patients who have diabetes when consumed in the acceptable daily intake levels established by the U.S. Food and Drug Administration. Whether nonnutritive sweeteners improve long-term glycemic control or assist in weight loss is known.

Protein

Protein accounts for 15% to 20% of daily energy intake. In individuals who have controlled type 2 diabetes, ingested protein does not increase plasma glucose concentration, although ingested protein is as potent a stimulus of insulin secretion as carbohydrate [11,28]. No evidence suggests that usual protein intake should be modified if renal function is normal [29].

For diabetic patients who have less-than-optimal glycemic control, protein requirements may be greater than recommended daily allowance, but not greater than 20% of daily energy intake. Available evidence suggests that the dietary protein does not slow the absorption of carbohydrate, and that dietary protein and carbohydrate do not take longer to raise plasma glucose than carbohydrate alone, and therefore do not prevent late-onset hypoglycemia.

Dietary fat

Less than 10% of energy intake should be derived from dietary fat, with cholesterol intake less than 300 mg/d. Intake of trans fatty acids should be minimized.

Incorporating two to three servings of plant stanols and sterols into the daily diet will decrease total and low-density lipoprotein cholesterol. Two or more servings of fish per week provide omega3 polyunsaturated fat.

Fat intake should be individualized and designed to fit ethnic and cultural backgrounds.

Micronutrients

Restricting sodium intake to less than 2 g/d may cause older individuals who enjoy salty foods to further limit their caloric intake and increase their risk for nutritional deficiencies. Older subjects are more likely to have deficiencies in micronutrients, such as thiamine, vitamin B_{12}, folate, vitamin C, vitamin D, calcium, zinc, and magnesium [30]. All older adults should be advised to have a calcium intake of at least 1500 mg/d [31].

The Baltimore longitudinal study of aging found that daily intake and plasma levels of certain antioxidants such as vitamin A and vitamin E were suboptimal in the elderly population [32]. In the Framingham study, poor intake of folate, vitamin B_6, and vitamin B_{12} was related to increased plasma homocysteine concentration and increased prevalence of carotid stenosis [33].

In a study in healthy elderly subjects supplemented with chromium 1000 μg/d, chromium did not alter insulin sensitivity, lipid profile, or body composition [34,35]. High-dose vitamin E supplementation has been associated with increased mortality [36]. Vitamins E and C interfere with the ability to measure glucose [37].

Vitamin D levels fall longitudinally as people age [38]. Vitamin D deficiency has been found in more than 50% of nursing home residents, with 15% to 20% of these having evidence of secondary hyperparathyroidism [39–41].

A meta-analysis of vitamin D replacement found it to be associated with decreased mortality [42]. Daily supplementation with 1000 mg of elemental calcium and 800 IU of vitamin D seems safe and decreases the risk for osteoporosis. However, a recent randomized study of 1471 postmenopausal women found that 1 g of calcium daily resulted in increased cardiovascular events [43].

Nutritional supplements are appropriate when patients cannot meet nutritional needs through diet. Dietary supplement use occurred in more than 50% of subjects in the National Health and Nutrition Examination Survey and was associated with lower risk for prevalent elevated blood pressure and diabetes [44].

Trace minerals

Hypomagnesemia occurs in 13.5% to 47.7% of patients who have diabetes mellitus [45]. It is more common when diabetic control is poor [46]. Even patients who have diabetes and normomagnesemia have a intracellular magnesium deficiency [47]. Insulin significantly lowers magnesium, whereas metformin increases it.

Hypomagnesemia is more common in patients who have diabetes who have retinopathy and hypertension [48]. Hypomagnesemia also independently predicts depression in older persons who have diabetes [49]. In patients who have diabetes, low serum magnesium is associated with increased all-cause mortality [50].

Zinc is an essential micronutrient that is a cofactor for more than 300 enzymes and stabilizes the structure of thousands of proteins. Zinc deficiency occurs in approximately 12% of older patients who have diabetes [51,52]. Zinc plays a role in insulin secretion, and zinc release from islet beta cells results in beta cell apoptosis in the presence of hyperinsulinemia [53].

Like magnesium tissue, zinc is decreased more than serum zinc [54]. Zinc deficiency in individuals who have diabetes is caused by hyperzincuria and zinc malabsorption [52,55]. Low serum zinc levels are associated with increased risk for both fatal and non-fatal cardiovascular events [56]. Zinc replacement reduces cholesterol and triglycerides [57], but supplementation has not been shown to improve diabetic control [52,58]. However, some evidence shows that zinc supplementation may improve immune function [59,60].

Selenium is an essential nutrient that protects against oxidative damage through selenium-dependent glutathione peroxidase. Seleno-proteins are also involved in immune function and thyroid function. More than 1% of the United States population take selenium supplements [61]. The National Prevention of Cancer Study found that people receiving a 200 µg supplement of selenium for 7.7 years had an increased risk for developing diabetes mellitus, with a hazard ratio of 2.70 (1.30–5.61) [62].

Plasma copper levels are elevated in persons who have type 2 diabetes mellitus [63]. Elevated copper levels are associated with the metabolic syndrome [64]. Elevated copper levels in the lens of patients who have diabetes may play a role in the accelerated development of cataracts that occurs with diabetes [65]. Increased copper levels in the aorta result in increased oxidative stress, which has been implicated in the pathogenesis of abdominal aortic aneurysms [66].

Alcohol intake

The European Prospective Investigation into Cancer in Norfolk study showed that consuming only up to 14 alcoholic beverages per week, not smoking, eating five servings of vegetables and fruits daily, and exercise improve physiologic age by 14 years in older persons [67].

Abstention from alcohol should be advised for women during pregnancy and for people who have medical problems, such as pancreatitis, advanced neuropathy, severe hypertriglyceridemia, or alcohol abuse. If individuals choose to drink alcohol, no more than two alcoholic beverages for adult men and no more than one drink for adult women are recommended per day. One alcoholic beverage is commonly defined as 12 oz of beer, 5 oz of wine, or 1.5 oz of distilled spirits, each of which contains 15 g of alcohol. Alcohol can have both hypoglycemic and hyperglycemic effects in people who have diabetes. To reduce risk for hypoglycemia, alcohol should be consumed with food.

Probiotics

Probiotics are live microorganisms that confer a health benefit in the host when given in sufficient quantities. They are mainly lactic acid bacilli, which convert carbohydrates into lactic acid. The most common strains are *Lactobacillus* and *Bifidobacterium*. Probiotics regulate the immune response [68]. They relieve diarrhea (rotavirus and *Clostridium difficile*), modulate lactose intolerance, and may improve constipation and other bowel disorders. A low-fat diet supplemented with *L acidophilus* and *L casei* delayed the onset of hyperglycemia and oxidative stress in rats fed a high fructose diet [69].

Prebiotics are nondigestible food ingredients that beneficially affect the host through selectively stimulating the growth or activity of bacteria that act as probiotics. Prebiotic foods include jicama, chicory, barley, and Jerusalem artichoke. These foodstuffs contain insulin and oligofructosaccharides. A nutritional supplement with oligosaccharides decreased mRNA for tumor necrosis factor alpha and interleukin-6 and decreased levels of sCD14, a substance shed by activated macrophages [70].

Fish oils

Fish oils are polyunsaturated omega-3 fatty acids, such as eicosapentaenoic acid and docosahexanoic acid. Epidemiologic studies have suggested that fish consumption is associated with a reduced risk for diabetes and glucose intolerance [71,72]. Omega-3 fatty acids reduce triglycerides and platelet reactivity in persons who have diabetes [73]. Some evidence shows that these compounds may enhance insulin sensitivity, although this is controversial [74,75].

The GISSI-Prevenzione trial found that 1 g/d of omega-3 fatty acids reduced death, nonfatal myocardial infarction, and stroke [76], perhaps because of an antiarrhythmic effect [77]. In 18,645 Japanese subjects receiving a statin, the addition of 1.8 g/d of eicosapentaenoic acid over 4.6 years reduced major coronary events [78]. Another study suggested omega-3 fatty acids promote plaque stability [79].

Physical activity

Exercise training can significantly slow the decline in maximal aerobic capacity that occurs with age, improve risk factors for atherosclerosis, slow the decline in age-related lean body mass, decrease central adiposity, and improve insulin sensitivity [80,81]. However, because of the potential risks of exercise (eg, cardiac ischemia, musculoskeletal, foot injuries, hypoglycemia) in patients treated with insulin, evaluation and education should occur before an exercise training program is initiated. Physical activity should increase gradually, and appropriate stretching, warm-up, and cooldown periods should accompany all exercises.

Summary

MNT for people who have diabetes should be individualized and taking into account an individual's usual food and eating habits, metabolic profile, treatment goals, and desired outcomes. Metabolic parameters, including glucose, HbA1c, lipids, blood pressure, body weight, and renal function (when appropriate), and quality of life must be monitored to assess the need for changes in therapy and ensure successful outcomes.

Ongoing nutrition self-management education and care must be available for individuals who have diabetes. Many areas of nutrition and diabetes require additional research, especially in the elderly population. The Diabetes Prevention Program showed that lifestyle modification, but not metformin, prevented diabetes in persons up to 85 years of age [82].

References

[1] Mazza AD, Morley JE. Update on diabetes in the elderly and the application of current therapeutics. J Am Med Dir Assoc 2007;8(8):489–92.

[2] Kim MJ, Rolland Y, Cepeda O, et al. Diabetes mellitus in older men. Aging Male 2006;9(3): 139–47.

[3] Diabetes Control and Complications Trial Research Group. The effect of intensive treatment of diabetes on the development and progression of long-term complications in insulin-dependent diabetes mellitus. N Engl J Med 1993;329(14):977–86.

[4] U.K. Prospective Diabetes Study (UKPDS) Group. Intensive blood-glucose control with sulphonylureas or insulin compared with conventional treatment and risk of complications in patients with type 2 diabetes. Lancet 1998;352(9141):837–53.

[5] American Diabetes Association special report: principles of nutrition and dietary recommendations for patients with diabetes mellitus: 1971. Diabetes 1971;20(9):633–4.

[6] American Diabetes Association: standards of medical care for patients with diabetes mellitus (position statement). Diabetes Care 2003;26(Suppl 1):S33–50.

[7] Mooradian AD. Biology of aging. In: Felsenthal G, Garrison SJ, Steinberg FU, editors. Rehabilitation of the aging and elderly patient. Baltimore (MD): Williams & Wilkins; 1994. p. 3–10.

[8] Morley JE. Weight loss in the nursing home. J Am Med Dir Assoc 2007;8(4):201–4.

[9] Thomas DR, Ashmen W, Morley JE, et al. Nutritional management in long-term care: development of a clinical guideline. Council for nutritional strategies in long-term care. J Gerontol A Biol Sci Med Sci 2000;55(12):M725–34.

[10] Morais JA, Gougeon R, Pencharz PB, et al. Whole body protein turnover in the healthy elderly. Am J Clin Nutr 1997;66(4):880–9.

[11] Gougeon R, Pencharz PB, Sigal RJ. Effect of glycemic control on the kinetics of whole-body protein metabolism in obese subjects with non-insulin dependent diabetes mellitus during iso and hypoenergetic feeding. Am J Clin Nutr 1997;65(3):861–70.

[12] Rosenthal MJ, Fajardo M, Gilmore S, et al. Hospitalization and mortality of diabetes in older adults. A 3-year prospective study. Diabetes Care 1998;21(2):231–5.

[13] Rodriguez-Saldana J, Morley JE, Reynoso MT, et al. Diabetes mellitus in a subgroup of older Mexicans: prevalence, association with cardiovascular risk factors, functional and cognitive impairment, and mortality. J Am Geriatr Soc 2002;50(1):111–6.

[14] Morley JE. Weight loss in older persons: new therapeutic approaches. Curr Pharm Des 2007; 13(35):3637–47.

[15] Wedick NM, Barrett-Connor E, Knoke JD, et al. The relationship between weight loss and all-cause mortality in older men and women with and without diabetes mellitus: the Rancho Bernardo Study. J Am Geriatr Soc 2002;50(11):1810–5.

[16] Visser M, Deurenberg P, Van Staveren WA, et al. Resting metabolic rate and diet-induced thermogenesis in young and elderly subjects: relationship with body composition, fat distribution, and physical activity level. Am J Clin Nutr 1995;61(4):772–8.

[17] Roberts SB, Fuss P, Heyman MB, et al. Influence of age on energy requirements. Am J Clin Nutr 1995;62(5 Suppl):1053S–8S.

[18] Morley JE. Is weight loss harmful to older men? Aging Male 2006;9(3):135–7.

[19] Chapman IM, MacIntosh CG, Morley JE, et al. The anorexia of ageing. Biogerontology 2002;3(1–2):67–71.

[20] Mooradian AD, McLaughlin S, Boyer CC, et al. Diabetes care for older adults. Diabetes Spectrum 1999;12:70–7.

[21] Tariq SH, Karcic E, Thomas DR, et al. The use of no concentrated sweets diet in the management of type 2 diabetes in the nursing home. J Am Diet Assoc 2001;101(12):1463–6.

[22] Coulston AM, Mandelbaum D, Reaven GM. Dietary management of nursing home residents with non-insulin dependent diabetes mellitus. Am J Clin Nutr 1990;51(1):62–71.

[23] American Diabetes Association. Translation of the diabetes nutrition recommendations for health care institutions. Diabetes Care 2002;25(Suppl 1):S61–3.

[24] Riccardi G, Rivellese A, Pacioni D, et al. Separate influence of dietary carbohydrate and fibre on the metabolic control in diabetes. Diabetologia 1984;26(2):116–21.

[25] Giacco R, Parillo M, Rivellese AA, et al. Long-term dietary treatment with increased amounts of fiber-rich low-glycemic index natural food improves blood glucose control and reduces the number of hypoglycemic events in type 1 patients with diabetes. Diabetes Care 2000;23(10):1461–6.

[26] Mooradian AD, Osterweil D, Petrasek D, et al. Diabetes mellitus in elderly nursing home patients: a survey of clinical characteristics and management. J Am Geriatr Soc 1988;36(5):391–6.

[27] Malerbi DA, Paiva ES, Duarte AL, et al. Metabolic effects of dietary sucrose and fructose in type 2 diabetic subjects. Diabetes Care 1996;19(11):1249–56.

[28] Millward DJ, Fereday A, Gibson N, et al. Aging, protein requirements and protein turnover. Am J Clin Nutr 1997;66(4):774–86.

[29] Brodsky IG, Robbins DC, Hiser E, et al. Effects of low-protein diets on protein metabolism in insulin-dependent diabetes mellitus patients with early nephropathy. J Clin Endocrinol Metab 1992;75(2):351–7.

[30] Koehler KM, Pareo-Tubbeh SL, Romero LJ, et al. Folate nutrition and older adults: challenges and opportunities. J Am Diet Assoc 1997;97(2):167–73.

[31] Kinyamu HK, Gallagher JC, Balhorn KE, et al. Serum vitamin D metabolites and calcium absorption in normal young and elderly free living women and women living in nursing homes. Am J Clin Nutr 1991;65(3):790–7.

[32] Volkert D, Kruse W, Oster P, et al. Malnutrition in geriatric patients: diagnostic and prognostic significance of nutritional parameters. Ann Nutr Metab 1991;36(2):97–112.

[33] Selhub J, Jacques PF, Wilson PW, et al. Vitamin status and intake as primary determinants of homocysteinemia in an elderly population. JAMA 1993;270(22):2693–8.

[34] Amato P, Morales AJ, Yen SSC. Effects of chromium picolinate supplementation on insulin sensitivity, serum lipids, and body composition in healthy, nonobese older men and women. J Gerontol A Biol Sci Med Sci 2000;55(5):M250–63.

[35] Jain SK, McVie R, Jaramillo JJ, et al. Effect of modest vitamin E supplementation on glycated hemoglobin and triglyceride levels and red cell indices in type 1 diabetic patients. J Am Coll Nutr 1996;15(5):458–61.

[36] Bjelakovic G, Nikolova D, Gluud LL, et al. Mortality in randomized trials of antioxidant supplements for primary and secondary prevention: systemic review and meta-analysis. J Am Med Assoc 2007;297(8):842–57.

[37] Morley JE, Kaiser FE. Unique aspects of diabetes mellitus in the elderly. Clin Geriatr Med 1990;6(4):693–702.

[38] Perry HM 3rd, Horowitz M, Morley JE, et al. Longitudinal changes in serum 25-hydroxyvitamin D in older people. Metabolism 1999;48(8):1028–32.

[39] Drinka PJ, Krause PF, Nest LJ, et al. Determinants of parathyroid hormone levels in nursing home residents. J Am Med Dir Assoc 2007;8(5):328–31.

[40] Hamid Z, Riggs A, Spencer T, et al. Vitamin D deficiency in residents of academic long-term care facilities despite having been prescribed vitamin D. J Am Med Dir Assoc 2007;8(2):71–5.

[41] Morley JE. Should all long-term care residents receive vitamin D? J Am Med Dir Assoc 2007; 8(2):69–70.

[42] Autier P, Gandini S. Vitamin D supplementation and total mortality. Arch Intern Med 2007; 167(16):1730–7.

[43] Bolland MJ, Barber A, Doughty RN, et al. Vascular events in healthy older women receiving calcium supplementation: randomised controlled trial. BMJ 2008;336:1–8.

[44] Block G, Jensen CD, Norkus EP, et al. Usage patterns, health, and nutritional status of long-term multiple dietary supplement users: a cross-sectional study. Nutr J 2007;6:30.

[45] Pham PC, Pham PM, Pham SV, et al. Hypomagnesemia in patients with type 2 diabetes. Clin J Am Soc Nephrol 2007;2(2):366–73.

[46] Sales CH, Pedrosa LF. Magnesium and diabetes mellitus: their relation. Clin Nutr 2006; 25(4):554–62.

[47] Gorelik O, Efrati S, Berman S, et al. Effect of various clinical variables on total intracellular magnesium in hospitalized normomagnesemic diabetic patients before discharge. Biol Trace Elem Res 2007;120(1–3):102–9.

[48] Sharma A, Dabla S, Agrawal RP, et al. Serum magnesium: an early predictor of course and complications of diabetes mellitus. J Indian Med Assoc 2007;105(1):16–20.

[49] Barragan-Rodriguez L, Rodriguez-Moran M, Guerrero-Romero F. Depressive symptoms and hypomagnesemia in older diabetic subjects. Arch Med Res 2007;38(7):752–6.

[50] Haglin L, Tornkvist B, Backman L. Prediction of all-cause mortality in a patient population with hypertension and type 2 DM by using traditional risk factors and serum-phosphate, -calcium and -magnesium. Acta Diabetol 2007;44(3):138–43.

[51] Kinlaw WB, Levine AS, Morley JE, et al. Abnormal zinc metabolism in type II diabetes mellitus. Am J Med 1983;75(2):272–7.

[52] Niewoehner CB, Allen JI, Boosalis M, et al. Role of zinc supplementation in type II diabetes mellitus. Am J Med 1986;81(1):63–8.

[53] Devirgiliis C, Zalewski PD, Perozzi G, et al. Zinc fluxes and zinc transporter genes in chronic diseases. Science Digest 2007;622:84–93.

[54] Levine AS, McClain CJ, Handwerger BS, et al. Tissue zinc status of genetically diabetic and streptozotocin-induced diabetic mice. Am J Clin Nutr 1983;37(3):382–6.

[55] Cunningham JJ, Fu A, Mearkle PL, et al. Hyperzincuria in individuals with insulin-dependent diabetes mellitus: concurrent zinc status and the effect of high-dose zinc supplementation. Metabolism 1994;43(12):1558–62.

[56] Soinio M, Marneimi J, Laakso M, et al. Serum zinc level and coronary heart disease events in patients with type 2 diabetes. Diabetes Care 2007;30(3):523–8.

[57] Partida-Hernandez G, Arreola F, Fenton B, et al. Effect of zinc replacement on lipids and lipoproteins in type 2-diabetic patients. Biomed Pharmacother 2006;60(4):161–8.

[58] Beletate V, ElDib RP, Atallah AN. Zinc supplementation for the prevention of type 2 diabetes mellitus. Cochrane Database Syst Rev 2007;(1):CD005525.

[59] Mooradian AD, Norman DC, Morley JE. The effect of zinc status on the immune function of diabetic rats. Diabetologia 1988;31(9):703–7.

[60] Mooradian AD, Morley JE. Micronutrient status in diabetes mellitus. Am J Clin Nutr 1987; 45(5):877–95.

[61] Bleys J, Navas-Acien A, Guallar E. Selenium and diabetes: more bad news for supplements. Ann Intern Med 2007;147(4):271–2.

[62] Stranges S, Marshall JR, Natarajan R, et al. Effects of long-term selenium supplementation on the incidence of type 2 diabetes. A randomized trial. Ann Intern Med 2007;147(4):217–23.

[63] Batista MN, Cuppari L, deFatima Campos Pedrosa L, et al. Effect of end-stage renal disease and diabetes on zinc and copper status. Biol Trace Elem Res 2006;112(1):1–12.

[64] Aguilar MV, Saavedra P, Arrieta FJ, et al. Plasma mineral content in type-2 diabetic patients and their association with the metabolic syndrome. Ann Nutr Metab 2007;51(5):402–6.

[65] Aydin E, Cumurcu T, Ozuguriu F, et al. Levels of iron, zinc, and copper in aqueous humor, lens, and serum in nondiabetic and diabetic patients: their relation to cataract. Biol Trace Elem Res 2005;108(1–3):33–41.

[66] Koksal C, Ercan M, Bozkurt AK, et al. Abdominal aortic aneurysm or aortic occlusive disease: role of trace element imbalance. Angiology 2007;58(2):191–5.

[67] Khaw KT, Wareham N, Bingham S, et al. Combined impact of health behaviours and mortality in men and women: the EPIC-Norfolk prospective population study. PLoS Med 2008;5(1):e12.

[68] Gill H, Prasad J. Probiotics, immunomodulation, and health benefits. Adv Exp Med Biol 2008;606:423–54.

[69] Yadav H, Jain S, Sinha PR. Antidiabetic effect of probiotic dahi containing Lactobacillus acidophilus and Lactobacillus casei in high fructose fed rats. Nutrition 2007;23(1):62–8.

[70] Schiffrin EJ, Thomas DR, Kumar VB, et al. Systemic inflammatory markers in older persons: the effect of oral nutritional supplementation with prebiotics. J Nutr Health Aging 2007;11(6):475–9.

[71] Feskens EJ, Virtanen SM, Rasanen L, et al. Dietary factors determining diabetes and impaired glucose tolerance. A 20-year follow-up of the Finish and Dutch cohorts of the Seven Countries Study. Diabetes Care 1995;18:1104–12.

[72] Raheja BS, Sadikot SM, Phatak RB, et al. Significance of the N-6/N-3 ratio for insulin action in diabetes. Ann N Y Acad Sci 1993;683:258–71.

[73] DeCaterina R, Madonna R, Bertolott A, et al. n-3 fatty acids in the treatment of diabetic patients. Biological rationale and clinical data. Diabetes Care 2007;30:1012–26.

[74] Rivellese AA, Maffettone A, Iovine C, et al. Long-term effects of fish oil on insulin resistance and plasma lipoproteins in NIDDM patients with hypertriglyceridemia. Diabetes Care 1996; 19(11):1207–13.

[75] Kabir M, Skurnik G, Naour N, et al. Treatment for 2 mo with n 3 polyunsaturated fatty acids reduces adiposity and some atherogenic factors but does not improve insulin sensitivity in women with type 2 diabetes: a randomized controlled study. Am J Clin Nutr 2007;86(6): 1670–9.

[76] Gruppo Italiano per lo Studio della Sopravvivenza nell'Infarcto miocardico: dietary supplementation with n-3 polyunsaturated fatty acids and vitamin E after myocardial infarction: results of the GISSI-Prevenzione trial. Lancet 1999;354:447–55.

[77] DeCaterina R, Madonna R, Zucchi R, et al. Antiarrhythmic effects of omega-3 fatty acids: From epidemiology to bedside. Am Heart J 2003;146:420–30.

[78] Yokoyama M, for the Japan EPA Lipid Intervention Study (JELIS). Effects of eicosapentaenoic acid (EPA) on major cardiovascular events in hypercholesterolemic patients. Circulation 2005;112:3362.

[79] Thies F, Garry JM, Yaqoob P, et al. Association of n-3 polyunsaturated fatty acids with stability of atherosclerotic plaques: a randomized controlled trial. Lancet 2003;361:477–85.

[80] Hagberg JM. Effect of training on the decline of Vo_{2max} with aging. Fed Proc 1987;46(5): 1830–3.

[81] LaCroix AZ, Leveille SG, Hecht JA, et al. Does walking decrease the risk of cardiovascular disease hospitalizations and death in older adults? J Am Geriatr Soc 1996;44(2):113–20.

[82] Crandall J, Schade D, Ma Y, et al. Diabetes Prevention Program Research Group. The influence of age on the effects of lifestyle modification and metformin in prevention of diabetes. J Gerontol A Biol Sci Med Sci 2006;61(10):1075–81.

CLINICS IN GERIATRIC MEDICINE

ELSEVIER
SAUNDERS

Clin Geriatr Med 24 (2008) 515–527

Eye Disease and the Older Diabetic

Nina Tumosa, PhD[a,b,*]

[a]Geriatrics Research, Education, and Clinical Center, St. Louis VA Medical Center,
St. Louis, MO 63125, USA
[b]Division of Geriatrics, Saint Louis University, 11G JB Geriatrics Research,
Education, and Clinical Center, St. Louis VA Medical Center,
St. Louis, MO 63125, USA

Multiple visual complications accompany diabetes mellitus (DM) of long duration. The most common complications include numerous ocular and periocular changes that characterize diabetic retinopathy. These changes are characterized by exudates, microaneurysms, hemorrhages, and, less frequently, neovascularization, all of which lead to a decrease in visual acuity and, perhaps, to blindness. Indeed, diabetic retinopathy is a leading cause of blindness in the industrialized world in people between the ages of 25 and 74 years [1] and is the fourth leading cause of blindness in people of all ages in developing countries [2]. Annually, between 12,000 and 24,000 diabetic patients in the United States become legally blind as a result of complications of diabetic retinopathy [3]. Moreover, every diabetic patient is at risk for even more changes to vision than those that occur as a result of DM.

The elderly diabetic patient is 1.5 times more likely to develop vision loss and blindness than is an age-matched nondiabetic person [4]. Just as age is a risk factor for developing multiple chronic medical conditions, so too is age a risk factor for developing multiple visual comorbidities. In addition to diabetic retinopathy, other relatively common eye conditions that increase in incidence with age include retinal detachment, vitreous hemorrhage, macular edema, retinal vein occlusion, macular degeneration, cataracts, and glaucoma. Indeed, cataracts, glaucoma and macular degeneration are four times more likely to cause vision loss and blindness than is diabetic retinopathy [5]. Therefore, older diabetic persons are vulnerable to developing decreasing visual abilities, and perhaps blindness, not only because of diabetic retinopathy but also because of its synergy with multiple other comorbid risk factors.

* 11G JB GRECC, St. Louis Veterans Administration Medical Center, St. Louis, MO 63125.
E-mail address: tumosan@slu.edu

0749-0690/08/$ - see front matter. Published by Elsevier Inc.
doi:10.1016/j.cger.2008.03.002

geriatric.theclinics.com

This article begins with the rather discouraging discussion of the multiple risk factors for low vision and blindness and the resulting disabilities that plague the aging diabetic patient. Conditions such as diabetic retinopathy, glaucoma, cataracts, dry eye syndrome, and macular degenerations are discussed, as are their resultant effects on the risk of falling, poor nutrition, infection rates, reduced physical activity, increased social isolation and depression, medication errors, hospitalizations, and mortality. It ends with a more optimistic discussion of current and future treatments for eye diseases in older diabetics that offer hope in the attenuation and prevention of vision loss and any consequential disability.

Visual consequences of diabetic retinopathy

Risk factors of diabetes mellitus

Many risk factors affect the rate at which diabetic retinopathy progresses. These risk factors include age [6,7], race [8–10], obesity [8], smoking [11], proteinuria [12], depression [13,14], dyslipidemia [11], duration of DM [6,7,9,10], cardiovascular diseases [15,16], uncontrolled systemic hypertension [9,11,12], parental history of DM [8], rapid glycemic control before cataract surgery [17], eating disorders [18], and poor glycemic control [6,19]. Although some of these risk factors cannot be controlled, many of them can be. The rate at which vision fails can be slowed with careful management and corporation between the patient and the health care team.

Clinical signs of diabetes mellitus

There are many clinical signs indicative of the presence of diabetic retinopathy (Table 1). The only sign that can be determined by the patient reliably without a comprehensive eye examination performed by an ophthalmologist or optometrist is decreased visual acuity, as evidenced by fluctuations in refractive error, distorted vision and/or blurred vision. A dilated fundus examination should be done to determine if these acuity changes are caused by retinal detachment, macula edema, vitreous or preretinal hemorrhage, or neovascularization of the disc or elsewhere. Less apt to be noticed by the patient are abnormalities in color vision and small visual field scotomas, which almost always are documented for the first time during an eye examination. Other signs of diabetic retinopathy that can be confirmed with an eye examination are hard exudates, cotton wool spots, arteriolar narrowing, fibrotic proliferation, dot-, blot-, and flame-shaped hemorrhages, venous tortuosity and beading, microaneurysms, and intraretinal microvascular abnormalities. Because the eye examination is so critical to the confirmation of many of these changes, the American Diabetes Association's Clinical Practice Guidelines [20] for examining a patient who has diabetic retinopathy include performing (1) comprehensive eye examinations

Table 1
Common ocular and periocular manifestations of diabetes mellitus

Site or condition	Visual system consequences of diabetes mellitus
Refraction	Blurred vision
	Distorted vision
	Fluctuations in refractive error
Tear films	Dry eyes
Vitreous	Detachments
Macula	Maculopathy
	Ischemic
	Exudative
	Edematous
	Macula edema
Retina	Detachments
	Retinal edema
	Vein occlusions
	Micro aneurysms
	Artery occlusions
	Neovascularization
	Exudates (soft and hard)
	Intraretinal hemorrhages

within 3 to 5 years of the onset of DM in type 1 diabetics and immediately after initial diagnosis in type 2 diabetics; (2) subsequent annual dilated fundus examinations; (3) prompt referral to a retinal specialist of patients who have macular edema, severe nonproliferative diabetic retinopathy, or proliferative diabetic retinopathy; and (4) strict control of elevated blood pressure.

Visual consequences of common comorbid eye diseases

DM is a systemic disease. Therefore, it negatively affects nerves and cells throughout the body, not just in the visual system. As a consequence, other eye diseases also may be precipitated or exacerbated by DM. The most common and vision-threatening of those diseases are dry eye syndrome, cataracts, macular edema, neovascular glaucoma, and macular degeneration (Table 2).

Dry eye syndrome

Persons who have DM tend to develop dry eye syndrome [22–25]. This is especially true for women [26]. Diabetic patients who have dry eye syndrome have difficulty reading, working, using a computer, watching television, and driving [27]. The severity of dry eye syndrome is correlated with poor glycemic control and the duration of DM.

Cataracts

Research on the relationship between cataracts and DM is complicated, perhaps because both are age dependent and perhaps because there are so

Table 2
Comorbidities of diabetic retinopathy

Condition/disease	Location/manifestation
Neuropathies	Palsies of cranial nerves III, IV, and VI cause problems with the extraocular muscles
	Cranial nerve VII (Bell's palsy) affects the eyelids and leads to dry eye syndrome [21]
	Damage to cranial nerve II (Optic Nerve) leads to ischemic optic neuropathy and neovascularization of the disc
Glaucoma	Neovascularization of the iris
	Ganglion cell apoptosis blocks the trabecular network
Age-related macular degeneration	In patients who have macular degeneration, visual acuity declines earlier and more markedly in patients with diabetes than in those without diabetes
Cataracts	Lens: premature cortical cataracts and posterior subcapsular cataracts
Dry eye syndrome	Interrupted tear film layer, irritated corneas, corneal ulcers, abrasions, hypoesthesia, poor epithelial healing

many subclassifications of cataracts based on the location of the opacity in the lens. There is widespread agreement that diabetic persons are at risk of earlier presentation of subcapsular cataracts and other lens epithelial changes than are nondiabetic persons [28–31]. Therefore, persons who have DM need to be mindful of their glycemic control, especially as they age and their odds of developing cataracts increase.

As inconvenient as early presentation with cataracts is, a more serious concern for the diabetic patient is the increased risk for macula edema (a $\geq 30\%$ increase in the thickness of the macula) and poor visual results following cataract removal [32–34]. Postoperative macular edema is slightly more common in persons who have DM than in persons without DM, but it resolves spontaneously in persons who do not have DM and persists and/or worsens in those who have diabetic retinopathy. All diabetic patients need close observation for 3 to 6 months following cataract surgery, with an intervention of laser photocoagulation as required to prevent visual loss [35,36].

Neovascular glaucoma

Neovascular glaucoma has three clinical stages: (1) rubeosis iridis (formation of a fibrovascular membrane on the surface of the iris), (2) secondary open-angle glaucoma, and (3) synechia of the iris causing angle-closure glaucoma with a corresponding rise in intraocular pressure. Ganglion cell apoptosis also can lead to an increased incidence of open-angle glaucoma because of blockage of the trabecular network [37]. A third of the cases of neovascular glaucoma occur after proliferative diabetic retinopathy [38]. This condition is both painful and vision threatening. The most common treatments are medicines that are anti-inflammatory agents (steroids, cycloplegic agents) or that reduce the production of aqueous humor (carbonic anhydrase antagonists and beta-blockers), trabeculectomy (creating a fistula between the anterior chamber and the subconjunctival space) with antibiotics [39], or insertion of artificial drainage shunts. Given the poor outcomes for vision, neovascular glaucoma is a disease that should be monitored by a medical team that includes general practitioners, endocrinologists, neurologists, rheumatologists, and cardiologists [40]. Research on the development of strategies to increase the sensitivity of detecting the incidence of neovascular glaucoma is ongoing [41].

Macular degeneration

Although no causative effect has ever been found between age-related macular degeneration and DM, there nonetheless is an interaction. Both macular degeneration and the macula edema that results from diabetic retinopathy are associated with ocular neovascularization. A 10-year prospective study of 133 newly diagnosed diabetic patients and 144 nondiabetic controls who had macular degeneration found that visual acuity declines earlier and more markedly in diabetic patients than in control patients [42]. Interestingly, macular degeneration at baseline predicted the 10-year cardiovascular mortality, which was 4.7 times higher than in diabetic patients without macular degeneration. This increased mortality may result from a relationship between macular degeneration and atherosclerotic vascular disease caused by DM. Indeed, the recent successful treatment of both macular degeneration and macula edema with an antibody to vascular endothelial growth factor [43] suggests that they may have similar mechanisms of action on endothelial cells and vascular permeability. The current standard treatment of the retinal destruction caused by both macular degeneration and macular edema is thermal laser photocoagulation, which prevents further vision loss but does little to improve vision [44].

Macular edema

Macula edema is the primary mechanism of vision loss in diabetic retinopathy [45], presumably as a result of excess blood glucose that causes microvascular damage to the retina's extensive blood vessels. Laser photocoagulation is still the reference standard for treatment of clinically significant macular edema [46], but it rarely provides significant visual improvement. Vitreous surgery can improve visual acuity in about 50% of cases [47]. In an effort to find more efficacious treatments, several National Eye Institute clinical trials currently are investigating the effectiveness of various interventions to improve visual function, including laser photocoagulation [48], vitrectomy [49], anti-vascular endothelial growth factor (VEGF) plus laser photocoagulation [50], and anti-VEGF therapy alone [44], as well as a pilot study on peribulbar triamcinolone acetonide injections versus laser photocoagulation [51].

Consequences of vision loss in diabetics

In the United States, Medicare beneficiaries with vision loss incur six to 18 times more medical expenses than those without vision loss [52]. Most of those costs are not directly vision related. Twenty-seven percent to 41% of costs can be attributed to treatment for depression, injury, skilled nursing facility use, and long-term care admission. It is estimated that more than $2 billion in non–vision-related medical costs are paid by Medicare annually as a result of vision loss. The economic costs of vision loss among Americans ages 40 years and older is estimated to be about $35 billion dollars in direct medical costs, other direct costs, and lost productivity [53] plus $5 billion spent primarily on home care [54]. Four ocular diseases (macular degeneration, glaucoma, cataracts, and DM) account for about 75% of those expenses [53].

In addition to the great economic incentive for treating and managing vision loss aggressively in the diabetic patient, there is a social benefit from increased productivity and decreased disability. Vision rehabilitation traditionally has been directed to patients who are blind or who have very low vision but, when directed to persons who have milder forms of disability, can improve quality of life significantly [55]. There is increasing evidence that vision loss caused by DM is associated with increased rates of falling [56–58], fractures [59], medication errors [60], ophthalmologic infections and emergencies [61], clinical depression [62–64] (although not with increased associated mortality with that depression [65]), and longer hospitalizations [55]. Vision rehabilitation earlier, rather than later, would decrease all these risk factors.

Assessments and treatments of vision loss caused by diabetic retinopathy and associated comorbid visual losses

The keys to minimizing vision loss resulting from diabetic retinopathy are rapid diagnosis and timely interventions to prevent vision loss [66]. The education of people who have DM plays a critical role in the management and treatment of DM and, therefore, of diabetic retinopathy and its associated vision loss. Screening plays an important role in the early detection of ocular damage and proactive intervention to prevent further vision loss [11], particularly for diabetic patients in long-term care facilities [67–69]. Screening for the retinal damage that is so prevalent in diabetic retinopathy is done commonly by assessing fundus photographs taken during a dilated fundus examination. Currently, however, fundus photographs taken in older persons with small pupil dilation often are of poor quality because of bilateral pupil constriction and the presence of cataracts. With ever-improving computer analysis, it eventually should become possible to extract quantitative data about diabetic lesions and vascular changes from photographs that currently are graded inadequately by physicians or trained technicians [70].

Until the technology for assessment improves significantly, however, the strict control of DM through the use of nutritional therapy, exercise, and drug treatment is absolutely essential to minimize vision loss in diabetic patients. For the past 20 years, the treatment of ocular and periocular changes that threaten to lead to vision loss has consisted of ever-improving surgical techniques within the eyeball to remove scar tissue and debris resulting from hemorrhages. Currently, promising new treatments using antibodies, growth factors, and steroids to decrease or reverse the progressive vision losses are being researched.

Nutritional treatment

Proper nutrition is an integral component in maintaining normal blood glucose levels. Both tobacco use and diet, particularly the consumption of fatty acids and dietary fiber, are associated significantly with the rate of progression of diabetic retinopathy and retinopathy-related risk factors [71]. Diets that achieve good metabolic control have resulted in excellent control of diabetic retinopathy [72]. The American Diabetes Association [73] recommends that such diets be individualized to the patient's diagnosis and treatment goals, taking into account eating habits and other lifestyle factors. This personalized approach requires a diet prescribed by a registered dietitian, but all members of the medical team must have updated nutritional knowledge to support the patient in adopting a healthy life style [74] and to be able to assess the value and appropriateness of reported diets [75].

Exercise therapy

Physical activity helps persons who have DM achieve metabolic goals [76]. Exercise helps with glycemic and blood pressure control. This control, in turn, delays both the onset and progression of diabetic retinopathy. Longitudinal studies indicate significant improvements in glucose metabolism with aerobic exercise training and with resistance training in middle-aged and older men and women [77]. Older adults who have type 2 DM have impaired mobility and reduced fitness; there is ongoing research to develop optimal exercise programs, but success often has been limited. A specially developed form of tai chi, although developed specifically for diabetic patients, may not have been of sufficient intensity, frequency, or duration to effect positive changes in many aspects of physiology or health status relevant to older people who have DM [78]. More research is necessary before specific exercise protocols can be identified for slowing the progression of diabetic retinopathy and its concomitant vision loss in the older diabetic person.

Surgical treatment

Until very recently there have been no drugs or chemicals that have shown promise in either slowing or reversing the vision loss caused by the progression of diabetic retinopathy. Since 1980, panretinal photocoagulation laser surgery has been used to treat macular edema [79] and the vitreous hemorrhages [80,81] that accompany proliferative diabetic retinopathy. Focal laser photocoagulation reduces the risk of moderate visual loss by 50% to 70% in eyes with macular edema. The laser procedures, however, lack efficacy in some patients, create patient discomfort, seldom are effective with a single treatment, constrict peripheral visual fields, decrease night vision, reduce near vision, reduce visual acuity, and create retinal damage and scarring. Early vitrectomy improves visual recovery in patients who have proliferative retinopathy with accompanying severe vitreous hemorrhage. Intravitreal injections of steroids can be used when conventional treatments have failed in eyes with persistent loss of vision. Currently, laser photocoagulation and vitrectomy remain the conventional management protocols for diabetic retinopathy [82].

Pharmacologic approaches

The ultimate goal of the treatment of diabetic retinopathy and its associated comorbid vision-threatening diseases is prevention and reversal of vision loss. Pharmacologic methods to achieve these goals traditionally have concentrated on producing strict metabolic control and tight blood pressure control and have reduced the risk of moderate and severe visual loss by 50% in patients who have severe nonproliferative and proliferative diabetic retinopathy [83]. That success still leaves half of the diabetic patients who are unable to control diabetic retinopathy and the concomitant vision loss using those methods. An active research agenda to develop and approve new pharmaceuticals that will better protect visual acuity, macular thickness and, therefore, patient quality of life is currently underway.

Many new studies on the treatment of diabetic retinopathy have been based on the observations that microvascular damage in patients who have chronic hyperglycemia is mediated by interrelated pathways involving aldose reductase, advanced glycation end products, protein kinase C, and VEGF. Thus, a variety of promising new therapies targeting pathways that cause microvascular damage are under investigation for diabetic retinopathy [83,84]. Many of these therapies involve direct growth factor modulators including VEGF inhibitors, protein kinase C inhibitors, and steroids. Current research studies involving human subjects include a combination of panretinal photocoagulation and intravitreal injections of triamcinolone acetonide [85,86] to treat proliferative diabetic retinopathy; intravitreal injections of antibodies against VEGF to treat diabetic edema [87,88]; and the use of antibodies against VEGF, growth factors, and steroids to treat neovascularization [44]. All these studies are underway currently, and no specific treatment recommendations have yet been made. More comprehensive evaluations in multicenter, randomized, controlled clinical trials with longer follow-up are needed before clinical guidelines can be developed.

Summary

Early detection, constant surveillance, and aggressive treatment with exercise, diet, surgery, and pharmaceuticals to maintain tight glycemic and blood pressure control are the watchwords for minimizing vision loss in the diabetic patient. Clear, culturally appropriate patient education materials that provide information about DM, promote self-efficacy, and motivate self-care behaviors related to glycemic control are critical to the successful execution of this treatment plan [89,90]. Personal control over one's own health care has been shown to improve control of DM for patients who were taught to self-monitor their blood glucose levels [91]. All health care providers need to give consistent information, so there must be coordination of educational materials and of the message given to the patient. Educational tools such as reminder cards, informational brochures, self-care assessments, lists of available diabetes services, and daily recording sheets all enhance patient health literacy and compliance.

This consistent, culturally sensitive, educational approach is particularly important for the elderly patient who has diabetic retinopathy [92], because the disease has the potential to progress to visual disability and/or blindness. Visual loss has a large impact on the quality of life of an older person, because it contributes to morbidity and also to mortality [16,92–94]. If the patient wishes to address the DM actively, the health care team should provide the educational materials that will assist in that goal. If the loss of sight is not a priority, the team must respect that decision as well. Only through education and communication can the entire health care team, which includes the patient and the family as well as the health care providers, make the appropriate health care decisions to treat the entire patient, not just a single disease.

References

[1] National Institutes of Health. Available at: www.nei.nih.gov/eyedatap. Accessed December 23, 2007.

[2] World Health Organization. Available at: http://www.who.int/mediacentre/factsheets/fs282/en/accessed. Accessed December 25, 2007.

[3] Wild S, Roglic G, Green A, et al. Global prevalence of diabetes: estimates for the year 2000 and projections for 2030. Diabetes Care 2004;27(5):1047–53.

[4] Sinclair AJ, Bayer AJ, Girling AJ, et al. Older adults, diabetes mellitus and visual acuity: a community-based case-control study. Age Ageing 2000;29:335–9.

[5] Idil A, Caliskan D, Ocaktan E. The prevalence of blindness and low vision in older onset diabetes mellitus and associated factors: a community-based study. Eur J Ophthalmol 2004;14:298–305.

[6] Cikamatana L, Mitchell P, Rochtchina E, et al. Five-year incidence and progression of diabetic retinopathy in a defined older population: the Blue Mountains Eye Study. Eye 2007;21(4):465–71.

[7] Roy MS. Diabetic retinopathy in African Americans with type 1 diabetes: the New Jersey 725: I. Methodology, population, frequency of retinopathy, and visual impairment. Arch Ophthalmol 2000;118(1):97–104.

[8] Harris MI, Hadden WC, Knowler WC, et al. Prevalence of diabetes and impaired glucose tolerance and plasma glucose levels in U.S. population aged 20–74 yr. Diabetes 1987; 36(4):523–34.

[9] Roy MS, Affouf M. Six-year progression of retinopathy and associated risk factors in African American patients with type 1 diabetes mellitus: the New Jersey 725. Arch Ophthalmol 2006;124(9):1297–306.

[10] Varma R, Torres M, Pena F, et al, Los Angeles Latino eye study. Prevalence of diabetic retinopathy in adult Latinos: the Los Angeles Latino eye study. Ophthalmology 2004; 111(7):1298–306.

[11] Bloomgarden ZT. Screening for and managing diabetic retinopathy: current approaches. Am J Health Syst Pharm 2007;64(12 Suppl 12):S8–14.

[12] Klein R, Klein BE, Moss SE, et al. The Wisconsin Epidemiologic Study of Diabetic Retinopathy: XVII. The 14-year incidence and progression of diabetic retinopathy and associated risk factors in type I diabetes. Ophthalmology 1998;105(10):1801–15.

[13] Anderson D, Horton C, O'Toole M. Integrating depression care with diabetes care in real-world settings: lessons from the Robert Wood Johnson Foundation Diabetes Initiative. Diabetes Spectrum 2007;20:10–6.

[14] Roy MS, Peng B, Roy A. Risk factors for coronary disease and stroke in previously hospitalized African-Americans with type 1 diabetes: a 6-year follow-up. Diabet Med 2007;24(12): 1361–8.

[15] Juutilainen A, Lehto S, Ronnemaa T, et al. Retinopathy predicts cardiovascular mortality in type 2 diabetic men and women. Diabetes Care 2007;30(2):292–9.

[16] Lovestam-Adrian M, Hansson-Lundblad C, Torffvit O. Sight-threatening retinopathy is associated with lower mortality in type 2 diabetic subjects: a 10-year observation study. Diabetes Res Clin Pract 2007;77(1):141–7.

[17] Suto C, Hori S, Kato S, et al. Effect of perioperative glycemic control in progression of diabetic retinopathy and maculopathy. Arch Ophthalmol 2006;124(1):38–45.

[18] Rodin G, Olmsted MP, Rydall AC, et al. Eating disorders in young women with type 1 diabetes mellitus. J Psychosom Res 2002;53(4):943–9.

[19] Mitchell P, Smith W, Wang JJ, et al. Prevalence of diabetic retinopathy in an older community. The Blue Mountain Study. Ophthalmology 1998;105(3):406–11.

[20] The American Diabetes Association's Clinical Practice Guidelines. Available at: http://diabetes.org/for-health-professionals-and-scientists/cpr.jsp. Accessed October 27, 2007.

[21] Tiemstra JD, Khatkhate N. Bell's palsy: diagnosis and management. Am Fam Physician 2007;76(7):997–1002.

[22] Kaiserman I, Kaiserman N, Nakar S, et al. Dry eye in diabetic patients. Am J Ophthalmol 2005;139(3):498–503.

[23] Li HY, Pang GX, Xu ZZ. [Tear film function of patients with type 2 diabetes]. Zhongguo Yi Xue Ke Xue Yuan Xue Bao 2004;26(6):682–6 [in Chinese].

[24] Seifart U, Strempel I. [The dry eye and diabetes mellitus]. Ophthalmologie 1994;91(2):235–9 [in German].

[25] Yoon KC, Im SK, Seo MS. Changes in tear film and ocular surfaces in diabetes mellitus. Korean J Ophthalmol 2004;18(2):168–74.

[26] Sendecka M, Baryluk A, Polz-Dacewicz M. [Prevalence and risk factors of dry eye syndrome]. Przegl Epidemiol 2004;58(1):227–33 [in Polish].

[27] Mijanovic B, Dana R, Sullivan DA, et al. Impact of dry eye syndrome on vision-related quality of life. Am J Ophthalmol 2007;143(3):409–15.

[28] Klein BE, Klein R, Lee KE. Diabetes, cardiovascular disease, selected cardiovascular disease risk factors, and the 5-year incidence of age-related cataract and progression of lens opacities: the Beaver Dam Eye Study. Am J Ophthalmol 1998;126(6):782–90.

[29] Rowe NG, Mitchell PG, Cumming RG, et al. Diabetes, fasting blood glucose and age-related cataract: the Blue Mountains Eye Study. Ophthalmic Epidemiol 2000;7(2): 103–14.

[30] Struck HG, Heider C, Lautenschlager C. [Is diabetes in the elderly patient a risk factor for cataracts?]. Ophthalmologe 2001;98(7):952–65 [in German].

[31] Tkachov SI, Lautenschlager C, Ehrich D, et al. Changes in the lens epithelium with respect to cataractogenesis: light microscopic and Scheimpflug densitometric analysis of the cataractous and the clear lens of diabetics and non-diabetics. Graefes Arch Clin Exp Ophthalmol 2006;244(5):596–602.

[32] Chew EY, Benson WE, Remaley NA, et al. Results after lens extraction in patients with diabetic retinopathy: early treatment diabetic retinopathy study report number 25. Arch Ophthalmol 1999;117(12):1600–6.

[33] Krepler K, Biowski R, Schrey S, et al. Cataract surgery in patients with diabetic retinopathy: visual outcome, progression of diabetic retinopathy, and incidence of diabetic macular oedema. Graefes Arch Clin Exp Ophthalmol 2002;240(9):735–8.

[34] Parness R, Kleinman G, Katz H, et al. [Diabetic retinopathy following cataract surgery]. Harefuah 2005;144(11):763–7 [in Hebrew].

[35] Gupta A, Gupta V. Diabetic maculopathy and cataract surgery. Ophthalmol Clin North Am 2001;14(4):625–37.

[36] Kim SJ, Equi R, Bressler NM. Analysis of macula edema after cataract surgery in patients with diabetes using optical coherence tomography. Ophthalmology 2007;114(5):881–9.

[37] Nakamura M, Kanamori A, Negi A. Diabetes mellitus as a risk factor for glaucomatous optic neuropathy. Ophthalmologica 2005;219(1):1–10.

[38] Vancea PP, Abu-Taleb A. [Current trends in neovascular glaucoma treatment]. Rev Med Chir Soc Med Nat Iasi 2005;109(2):264–9 [in Romanian].

[39] Kiuchi Y, Sugimoto R, Nakae K, et al. Trabeculectomy with mitomycin C for treatment of neovascular glaucoma in diabetic patients. Ophthalmologica 2006;220(6):383–6.

[40] Konareva-Kostianeva M. Neovascular glaucoma. Folia Med (Plovdiv) 2005;47(2):5–11.

[41] Pasquale LR, Asefzadeh B, Dunphy RW, et al, Ocular TeleHealth Team. Detection of glaucoma-like optic discs in a diabetes teleretinal program. Optometry 2007;78(12): 657–63.

[42] Voutilainen-Kaunisto RM, Terasvirta ME, Uusitupa MI, et al. Age-related macular degeneration in newly diagnosed type 2 diabetic patients and control subjects. Diabetes Care 2000; 23(11):1672–8.

[43] Ng EW, Adamis AP. Anti-VEGF aptamer (pegaptanib) therapy for ocular vascular diseases. Ann N Y Acad Sci 2006;1082:151–71.

[44] Emerson MV, Lauer AK. Emerging therapies for the treatment of neovascular age-related macular degeneration and diabetic macular edema. BioDrugs 2007;21(4):245–57.

[45] Davidson JA, Ciulla TA, McGill JB, et al. How the diabetic eye loses vision. Endocrine 2007; 31(1):107–16.

[46] Furiani BA, Meyer CH, Rodrigues EB, et al. Emerging pharmacologies for diabetic macular edema. Expert Opin Emerg Drugs 2007;12(4):591–603.

[47] Hatano N, Mizota A, Tanaka M. Vitreous surgery for diabetic macular edema—its prognosis and correlation between preoperative systemic and ocular conditions and visual outcomes. Ann Ophthalmol (Skokie) 2007;39(3):222–7.

[48] National Eye Institute. Clinical Studies Database: Diabetic Retinopathy Study Available at: www.nei.nih.gov/neitrials/viewStudyWeb.aspx?id=127. Accessed December 24, 2007.

[49] National Eye Institute. Clinical Studies Database: Diabetic Retinopathy Study Available at: www.nei.nih.gov/neitrials/viewStudyWeb.aspx?id=132. Accessed December 24, 2007.

[50] National Eye Institute. Clinical Studies Database: Diabetic Retinopathy Study Available at: www.nei.nih.gov/neitrials/viewStudyWeb.aspx?id=105. Accessed December 24, 2007.

[51] National Eye Institute. Clinical Studies Database: Diabetic Retinopathy Study Available at: www.nei.nih.gov/neitrials/viewStudyWeb.aspx?id=124. Accessed December 24, 2007.

[52] Javitt JC, Zhou Z, Willke RJ. Association between vision loss and higher medical care costs in Medicare beneficiaries' costs are greater for those with progressive vision loss. Ophthalmology 2007;114(2):238–45.

[53] Rein DB, Zhang P, Wirth KE, et al. The economic burden of major adult visual orders in the United States. Arch Ophthalmol 2006;124:1754–60.

[54] Frick KD, Gower EW, Kempen JH, et al. Economic impact of visual impairment and blindness in the United States. Arch Ophthalmol 2007;125:544–50.

[55] Jackson ML. Vision rehabilitation for Canadians with less that 20/40 acuity: the SmartSight model. Can J Ophthalmol 2006;41(3):355–61.

[56] Klein BE, Moss SE, Klein R, et al. Associations of visual function with physical outcomes and limitations 5 years later in an older population: the Beaver Dam eye study. Ophthalmology 2003;110(4):644–50.

[57] Strotmeyer ES, Cauley JA, Schwartz AV, et al. Nontraumatic fracture risk with diabetes mellitus and impaired fasting glucose in older white and black adults: the health, aging, and body composition study. Arch Intern Med 2005;165(14):1616–7.

[58] Schwartz AV, Vittinghoff E, Sellmeyer DE, et al, for the Health ABC Study. Diabetes-related complications, glycemic control, and falls in older adults. Diabetes Care 2008; 31(3):391–6.

[59] Ivers RQ, Cumming RG, Mitchell P, et al, for the Blue Mountain Eye Study. Diabetes and risk of fracture: the Blue Mountain Study. Diabetes Care 2001;24(7):1198–203.

[60] Windham BG, Griswold ME, Fried LP, et al. Impaired vision and the ability to take medications. J Am Geriatr Soc 2005;53(7):1179–90.

[61] Wipf JE, Paauw DS. Ophthalmologic emergencies in the patient with diabetes. Endocrinol Metab Clin North Am 2000;29(4):813–29.

[62] Flynn HW Jr, Chew EY, Simons BD, et al. Pars plana vitrectomy in the Early Treatment Diabetic Retinopathy Study. EDTRS report number 17. The Early Treatment Diabetic Retinopathy Study Research Group. Ophthalmology 1992;99(9):1351–7.

[63] Roy MS, Roy A, Affouf M. Depression is a risk factor for poor glycemic control and retinopathy in African-Americans with type 1 diabetes. Psychosom Med 2007;69(6):537–42.

[64] Talbot F, Nouwen A. A review of the relationship between depression and diabetes in adults. Is there a link? Diabetes Care 2000;23(10):1556–62.

[65] Freeman EE, Egleston BL, West SK, et al. Visual acuity change and mortality in older adults. Invest Ophthalmol Vis Sci 2005;46(11):4040–5.

[66] Klein BE, Klein R. Ocular problems in older Americans with diabetes. Clin Geriatr Med 1990;6(4):827–37.

[67] Mazza AD, Morley JE. Update on diabetes in the elderly and the application of current therapeutics. J Am Med Dir Assoc 2007;8(8):489–92.

[68] Hass LB. Optimizing insulin use in type 2 diabetes: role of basal and prandial insulin in long-term care facilities. J Am Med Dir Assoc 2007;8(8):502–10.

[69] Meyers RM, Broton JC, Woo-Rippe KW, et al. Variability in glycosylated hemoglobin values in diabetic patients living in long-term care facilities. J Am Med Dir Assoc 2007; 8(8):511–4.

[70] Sinclair SH. Diabetic retinopathy: the unmet needs for screening and a review of potential solutions. Expert Rev Med Devices 2006;3(3):301–13.

[71] Cundiff DK, Nigg CR. Diet and diabetic retinopathy: insights from the Diabetes Control and Complications Trial (DCCT). MedGenMed 2005;7(1):3.

[72] Hansson-Lundblad C, Agardh E, Agardh CD. Retinal examination intervals in diabetic patients on diet treatment only. Acta Ophthalmol Scand 1997;75(3):244–8.

[73] The American Diabetes Association. Nutrition recommendations and principles for people with diabetes mellitus. Diabetes Care 2004;23(Suppl 2):S43–6.

[74] Koura MR, Khairy AE, Abdel-Aal NM, et al. The role of primary health care in patient education for diabetes control. J Egypt Public Health Assoc 2001;76(3–4):241–64.

[75] Heller T, Maisios M, Shahar D. [Physicians' and nurses' knowledge and attitude towards nutritional therapy in diabetes]. Harefuah 2007;146(9):670–4 [in Hebrew].

[76] Franz MJ. Lifestyle modifications for diabetes management. Endocrinol Metab Clin North Am 1997;26(3):499–510.

[77] Ryan AS. Insulin resistance with aging: effects of diet and exercise. Sports Med 2000;30(5): 327–46.

[78] Tsang T, Orr R, Lam P, et al. Health benefits of Tai Chi for older patients with type 2 diabetes: the "Move It For Diabetes study"—a randomized controlled trial. Clin Interv Aging 2007;2(3):429–39.

[79] Writing Committee for the Diabetic Retinopathy Clinical Research Network, Fong DS, Strauber SF, et al. Comparison of the modified Early Treatment Diabetic Retinopathy Study and mild macular grid laser photocoagulation strategies for diabetic macular edema. Arch Ophthalmol 2007;125(4):469–80.

[80] Lovestam-Adrian M, Agardh CD, Torffvit O, et al. Type 1 diabetes patients with severe non-proliferative retinopathy may benefit from panretinal photocoagulation. Acta Ophthalmol Scand 2003;81(3):221–5.

[81] Luttrull JK, Musch DC, Spink CA. Subthreshold diode micropulse panretinal photocoagulation for proliferative diabetic retinopathy. Eye 2 February 9, 2007 [Epub ahead of print].

[82] Mohamed Q, Gillies MC, Wong TY. Management of diabetic retinopathy: a systematic review. JAMA 2007;298(8):902–16.

[83] Yam JC, Kwok AK. Update on the treatment of diabetic retinopathy. Hong Kong Med J 2007;13(1):46–60.

[84] Ryan GJ. New pharmacologic approaches to treating diabetic retinopathy. Am J Health Syst Pharm 2007;64(17 Suppl 12):S15–21.

[85] Choi KS, Chung JK, Lin SH. Laser photocoagulation combined with intravitreal triamcinolone acetonide injection in proliferative diabetic retinopathy with macular edema. Korean J Ophthalmol 2007;21(1):11–7.

[86] Zein WM, Noureddin BN, Jurdi FA, et al. Panretinal photocoagulation and intravitreal triamcinolone acetonide for the management of proliferative diabetic retinopathy with macular edema. Retina 2006;26(2):137–42.

[87] Arevalo JF, Fromow-Guerra J, Quiroz-Mercado H, et al, for the Pan-American Collaborative Retina Study Group. Primary intravitreal bevacizumab (Avastin) for diabetic macular edema: results from the Pan-American Collaborative Retina Study Group at 6-month follow-up. Ophthalmology 2007;114(4):743–50.

[88] Haritoglou C, Kook D, Neubauer A, et al. Intravitreal bevacizumab (Avastin) therapy for persistent diffuse diabetic macular edema. Retina 2006;26(9):999–1005.

[89] Heisler M, Smith DM, Hayward RA, et al. How well do patients' assessments of their diabetes self-management correlate with actual glycemic control and receipt of recommended diabetes services? Diabetes Care 2003;26(3):738–43.

[90] Heisler M, Piette JD, Spencer M, et al. The relationship between knowledge of recent HbA1c values and diabetes care understanding and self-management. Diabetes Care 2005;28(4): 816–22.

[91] Murata GH, Shah JH, Hoffman RM, et al. Diabetes Outcomes in Veterans Study (DOVES). Intensified blood glucose monitoring improves glycemic control in stable, insulin-treated veterans with type 2 diabetes: the Diabetes Outcomes in Veterans Study (DOVES). Diabetes Care 2003;26(6):1759–63.

[92] Massin P, Kaloustian E. The elderly diabetic's eyes. Diabetes Metab 2007;33(Suppl 1):S4–9.

[93] Hirai FE, Moss SE, Klein BE, et al. The relationship of glycemic control, exogenous insulin, and C-peptide levels to ischemic heart disease mortality over a 16-year period in persons with older-onset diabetes: Wisconsin Epidemiologic Study of Diabetic Retinopathy. Diabetes Care 2008;31(3):493–7.

[94] West SK, Munoz B, Istre J, et al. Mixed lens opacities and subsequent mortality. Arch Ophthalmol 2000;118(3):393–7.

ELSEVIER
SAUNDERS

CLINICS IN
GERIATRIC
MEDICINE

Clin Geriatr Med 24 (2008) 529–540

Anemia in Diabetic Patients

David R. Thomas, MD, FACP

Division of Geriatric Medicine, Saint Louis University Health Sciences Center,
1402 S. Grand Boulevard, Room M238, St. Louis, MO 63104, USA

The synthesis of blood components proceeds in the bone marrow in a complex, regulated manner. Anemia can be caused by failure of the bone marrow to produce adequate blood components (marrow failure), by blood loss from acute hemorrhage or chronic bleeding, or by a rapid breakdown of blood components (hemolysis) in the marrow or peripherally. The bone marrow can fail to produce adequate blood components because of primary impairment of hemoglobin synthesis (hemoglobinopathy), an altered maturation of blood cells (myelodysplastic syndromes), or inadequate nutrients (vitamin B_{12}, folate, pyridoxine, or iron) necessary for blood production.

The World Health Organization defines anemia as a hemoglobin concentration of less than 13 g/dL in men and less than 12 g/dL in women. Hemoglobin and hematocrit values differ little between the healthy elderly population and the younger population. Thus, anemia is not a normal finding in older persons, and hemoglobin concentration should not be adjusted downward in older persons [1,2].

Although little change in hemoglobin is observed with aging in healthy adults, the prevalence of anemia increases with each decade of life over the age of 70 years. In the established population data for adults aged 71 years or older, hemoglobin concentration was inversely associated with age. Nine percent of men and women aged 71 to 74 years were anemic. The proportion of anemic persons increased differentially with age, reaching 41% for men and 21% for women aged 90 years or older, respectively [3]. A similar trend was reported in the third National Health and Nutrition Examination Survey, in which the prevalence jumps from 11% in men aged 70 to 79 years to 22% in males aged 80 to 89 years [4]. Among 900 residents in 21 skilled nursing facilities, the prevalence of anemia was 48%, varying among facilities from 32% to 64%. Eleven percent of residents had a hemoglobin level of less than 100 g/L [5].

E-mail address: thomasdr@slu.edu

0749-0690/08/$ - see front matter © 2008 Elsevier Inc. All rights reserved.
doi:10.1016/j.cger.2008.03.003   *geriatric.theclinics.com*

The chief reason for this rise in both the incidence and the prevalence of ane-mia is the presence of comorbid conditions and gender-related changes with aging. Both anemia of chronic disease and anemia of chronic kidney disease increase with aging. Conceptually, anemia of chronic disease results from ab-normalities in iron distribution, including a blockage in the uptake and release of iron by erythrocytes, whereas anemia of renal disease is caused mainly by erythropoietin deficiency. The spectrum of disorders associated with anemia of chronic disease is broad and includes infectious, rheumatologic, and neo-plastic conditions and also disorders such as congestive heart failure. An indi-vidual can have anemia resulting from multiple causes, so careful diagnostic evaluation is required [6]. In particular, anemia caused by chronic disease and by chronic kidney frequently disease may co-exist in the same person [7].

There also is a marked gender difference in the frequency of anemia. In a population-based study, the corrected annual incidence of anemia was higher in men older than 65 years (90.3 per 1000 subjects) than in women older than 65 years (69.1 per 1000 subjects) [8]. Sex differences in hemoglobin concentra-tion result chiefly from differences in testosterone concentration. Hypogonad-ism in older males (andropause) commonly is associated with approximately a 1-g/dL fall in hemoglobin concentration [9]. Furthermore, men who have functional hypogonadism from pituitary adenomas are anemic [10], as are men undergoing therapy with total androgen blockade for prostate cancer [11].

The epidemiologic literature clearly demonstrates the link between ane-mia and frailty, functional impairment, mobility impairment, and falls in older persons [12–17]. Women who have a hemoglobin concentration be-tween 130 and 140 g/L have better mobility and lower mortality than those who have a hemoglobin concentration of less than 120 g/L [18]. Prolonged anemia results in left ventricular hypertrophy [19] and is strongly associated with an increased risk of subsequent myocardial infarction [20]. Among older persons who have congestive heart failure, the mortality risk is 34% higher with anemia [21] and increases by 1.6% for every 1% decrease in hematocrit [22]. Vascular dementia, but not Alzheimer's dementia, has been associated with anemia [23]. Quality of life is impaired in persons who have anemia, which produces a high level of fatigue [24,25].

Causes of anemia

Among 964 subjects older than 65 years enrolled in a Northern Italy pop-ulation study, the prevalence of anemia was 11% [26]. The causes of anemia included anemia of chronic disease (28.1%), iron deficiency anemia (16.7%), vitamin B_{12} and/or folate deficiency (10.5%), anemia of chronic kidney dis-ease (7.9%), and unexplained anemia (no evident cause for anemia, 36.8%).

An evaluation of 900 subjects in five skilled nursing facilities demon-strated a 48% prevalence of anemia [27]. One hundred subjects were selected randomly for a complete evaluation (excluding bone marrow examination), resulting in complete data for 60 subjects. Iron deficiency anemia was the most common cause (23%), followed by anemia of chronic disease (13%), chronic renal insufficiency (10%), presumed bone marrow failure/myelodysplasia (5%), hypothyroidism (2%), and a hemoglobinopathy (2%). No cause for the anemia was found in 45% of subjects (Fig. 1).

These and other studies confirm that the prevalence and etiology of anemia differ depending on the population studied. The data demonstrate, however, that iron deficiency anemia, anemia of chronic disease, and anemia of chronic kidney disease account for almost half of all anemia. Notably, unexplained anemia is the single largest category, accounting for a third to nearly half of all anemia. This unexplained anemia may result from limitations in epidemiologic studies. Complete evaluation of subjects who have anemia, including bone marrow examination, is rarely available in epidemiologic databases. For this reason, the presence of myelodysplasia syndromes or other explanations for anemia may be understated.

Anemia of chronic disease is the second most commonly diagnosed anemia after iron deficiency. The identification of hepcidin, an iron-regulated acute-phase protein, has shed light on the relationship of the immune response to iron homeostasis and anemia of chronic disease. Hepcidin expression is induced by lipopolysaccharide and interleukin-6 and is inhibited by tumor necrosis factor alpha [28]. The net effect is to produce decreased duodenal absorption of iron and the blocking of iron release from macrophages. Thus, anemia of chronic disease presents as anemia in the presence of adequate iron stores. Other proinflammatory cytokines, including interleukin-1 and tumor necrosis factor alpha, directly inhibit erythropoietin expression in vitro [29]. The severity of the anemia of chronic disease is related directly to the severity of the underlying chronic disease and the amount of circulating cytokines. Much higher amounts of erythropoietin are required to restore the formation of erythroid colony-forming units in the presence of high concentrations of interferon-gamma or tumor necrosis factor alpha [30].

The etiology of unexplained anemia is complex and remains largely a mystery. Artz and colleagues [27] demonstrated that after adjusting for

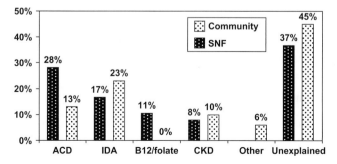

Fig. 1. Prevalence of anemia. ACD, anemia of chronic disease; CKD, anemia of chronic kidney disease; IDA, iron deficiency anemia; SNF, killed nursing facilities.

age, sex, and hemoglobin, erythropoietin levels were lower in subjects who had unexplained anemia than in those who had iron deficiency anemia, suggesting that erythropoietin may be an etiologic factor in unexplained anemia. These findings were confirmed by Ferruci and colleagues [26], who showed that iron deficiency anemia was associated with a high compensatory erythropoietin level, but anemia of chronic disease showed a bimodal erythropoietin response (low in some persons and high in others). Vitamin B_{12} and/or folate deficiency and unexplained anemia tended to be mild and showed little erythropoietin compensatory response. Indeed, erythropoietin levels in vitamin B_{12} deficiency and unexplained anemia were even lower than in non-anemic controls.

Ferruci and colleagues [26] found that subjects who had anemia of chronic disease had higher levels of interleukin-6 and C-reactive protein (but not tumor necrosis factor alpha) than seen in non-anemic controls. Subjects who had unexplained anemia had significantly lower C-reactive protein than non-anemic controls and had lower interleukin-6, tumor necrosis factor alpha, and C-reactive protein values than seen in any other type of anemia, suggesting that unexplained anemia is not related to inflammatory markers. Artz and colleagues [27] also found that interleukin-6 levels were markedly elevated in persons who had anemia of chronic disease but found no difference between the interleukin-6 levels seen in iron deficiency anemia and unexplained anemia. Unexplained anemia was characterized by low erythropoietin level, low levels of proinflammatory markers, and low lymphocyte counts, suggesting that the reduced erythropoietin response in unexplained anemia is not attributable to a proinflammatory state.

Anemia is strongly associated with chronic kidney disease because of the decreased production of erythropoietin by the kidney. For each 10-mL/min/ 1.73 m^2 decrease in estimated glomerular filtration rate, the hematocrit declined by 3.1%, and for every 1-mg/dL increase in serum creatinine, the hematocrit decreased 1.2% [31]. In a Health Maintenance Organization population with chronic renal insufficiency (creatinine > 1.2 mg/dL for female subjects and > 1.4 mg/dL for male subjects), 42% of subjects were anemic. Of the anemic subjects, 53% had hematocrit values below 30%, 31% of subjects had hematocrit values above 32.9%, and 16% had hematocrit values between 30% and 32.9% [32]. The development of anemia begins at relatively high levels of renal function (creatinine clearance of 60 mL/min in men and 40 mL/min in women) [33].

Anemia and diabetes

Diabetes has become the most common comorbid condition of end-stage renal disease in the United States [34]. Increased mortality has been associated with anemia and chronic kidney disease in diabetic subjects [35].

The prevalence of anemia in selected diabetic patients is approximately 13% to 15% and increases with duration of follow-up. After excluding subjects who had iron deficiency anemia, gastrointestinal bleeding, malignancy, anticoagulation therapy, or immunosuppressive therapy, 503 patients who had type 2 diabetes mellitus were followed for 5 years [36]. At baseline, 13% of subjects had anemia, although no individual had a baseline estimated glomerular filtration rate less than 30 mL/min. After 5 years, an additional 12% of subjects had developed anemia. As expected, the baseline presence of albuminuria, lower estimated glomerular filtration rate, and macrovascular complications predicted the development of anemia. After adjusting for these predictors, the subsequent development of anemia was not associated with gender, duration of diabetes, baseline hemoglobin level, C-reactive protein level, lipid level, blood pressure control, serum erythropoietin level, iron availability or stores, use of renin-angiotensin blockers, or thiazolidinediones.

Similar findings have been reported in persons who have type 1 diabetes [37]. In a clinic sample of 315 persons who had had type 1 diabetes for a mean duration of 20 years, 15% of women and 13% of men had anemia. The presence of albuminuria, stage 2 or greater chronic kidney disease, and macrovascular complications was strongly associated with the prevalence of anemia. Patients who had anemia were more than twice as likely to have established macrovascular disease (25%) than patients who did not have anemia (12%). More than half (56%) of all patients who had anemia had stage 2 or less chronic kidney disease, compared with less than 10% of patients with a normal hemoglobin. Overall, 69% of all patients who had anemia had either moderate renal impairment and/or elevated albuminuria. The prevalence of anemia was not associated with age, duration of diabetes, hemoglobin A1 c levels, or body mass index in this study.

These studies suggest that the pathway for the development of anemia in diabetic patients is related to the association between diabetes and chronic kidney disease. Persons who have diabetes, however, also are predisposed to develop other types of anemia, such as nutritional insufficiency or chronic disease, so a careful diagnostic approach is required.

Persons who have diabetes may have a specific predilection for the development of anemia other than chronic kidney disease. Anemia associated with chronic kidney disease is more common in patients who have diabetes than in patients who have chronic kidney disease of other etiologies [38]. Moreover, anemia occurs earlier in diabetic patients than in patients who have other types of chronic kidney diseases [39]. In addition, anemia often is found in diabetic patients without measurable renal impairment [40].

Treatment of anemia

The treatment of anemia is based on two principles. First, anemia can be deleterious in itself, requiring a compensatory increase in cardiac output to maintain systemic oxygen delivery. Second, anemia is associated with a poorer prognosis in a variety of conditions [41]. Therefore, moderate anemia warrants correction, especially in older patients and in those who have risk factors such as coronary artery disease, pulmonary disease, chronic kidney disease, or a combination of these factors.

Several diagnostic and treatment algorithms have been published [6,42,43]. Figs. 2–4 show schematic algorithms for diagnostic evaluation of anemia.

Iron deficiency anemia should be treated with iron replacement. The commonly used dose of ferrous sulfate is 325 mg, three times a day, providing 195 mg of elemental iron daily, and the treatment should last until the ferritin level is normalized. Various other iron replacement drugs differ in adverse effects and cost and may be considered in individual patients (Table 1). A reticulocyte count should be obtained 1 to 2 weeks after starting treatment with iron, and the lack of a response should prompt consideration of the use of intravenous iron. Intravenous iron therapy was associated with complications such as increased risk of bacteremia and infections in a subset of patients who had functional iron deficiency and high ferritin levels and who were receiving hemodialysis [41]. Other studies have not confirmed this risk of iron replacement, suggesting that iron is more likely to be absorbed and used by the erythron rather than by pathogens, as indicated by an increase in hemoglobin levels without demonstrable infectious complications [44]. Iron should be considered replaced when the serum ferritin concentration is maintained above 100 ng/mL. The level of serum ferritin above which patients will have iron overload is not known; however, a ceiling

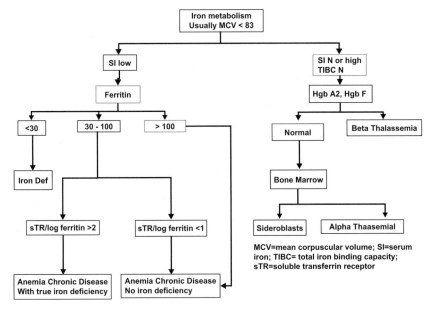

Fig. 2. Laboratory diagnosis of anemia. MCV, mean corpuscular volume; N, normal; SI, serum iron; sTR, soluble transferrin receptor; TIBC, total iron binding capacity.

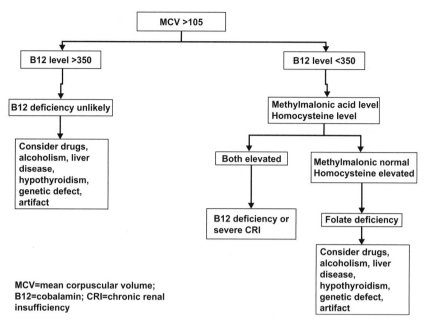

Fig. 3. Laboratory diagnosis of B_{12}/folate anemia. B_{12}, cobalamin; CRI, chronic renal insufficiency; MCV, mean corpuscular volume.

ferritin level of 800 ng/mL is suggested, and additional iron should not be administered once this value is reached [45].

Patients who have anemia of chronic disease and absolute iron deficiency demonstrated by a soluble transferrin receptor assay should receive supplemental iron therapy [44,46]. Iron supplementation also should be considered in patients who have anemia of chronic kidney disease who are unresponsive to therapy with erythropoietic agents because of iron deficiency.

Anemia caused by vitamin B_{12} deficiency is treated by vitamin B_{12} injections (1000 µg weekly for 1 month, then monthly thereafter), oral vitamin

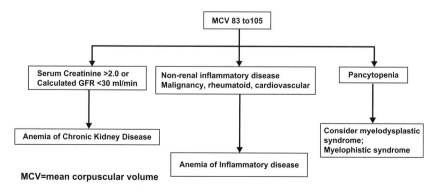

Fig. 4. Laboratory diagnosis of anemia. MCV, mean corpuscular volume.

Table 1
Comparison of iron replacement therapies

Iron preparations	Tablet size (mg)	Amount of elemental iron/pill (mg)	Number of pills required to provide approximately 200 mg elemental iron
Ferrous sulfate	325	65	3
Ferrous gluconate	325	38	5
Ferrous fumarate	200	66	3
Iron polysaccharide	150	150	2
Heme iron polypeptide	398	12	3–4

B_{12} (1000 μg daily, which should not be given with food), or intranasal vitamin B_{12}. Folic acid, 1 mg, should be used to treat folic acid deficiency and should be used during the first few weeks of vitamin B_{12} deficiency [47].

Although the usual dictum for managing anemia of chronic disease is to treat the underlying chronic illness, this approach often is unsatisfactory. Many of the chronic illnesses associated with anemia of chronic disease have limited and nonspecific treatments, and it may be difficult to determine which chronic illness to target. Erythropoietin therapy has been studied in patients who had anemia of chronic disease, although it is not approved by the Food and Drug Administration for this indication. Response rates were approximately 25% in myelodysplastic syndromes [48], 80% in multiple myeloma [49], and 95% in rheumatoid arthritis and chronic kidney disease [50]. Erythropoietin has been shown to increase hemoglobin concentration in patients who had anemia associated with surgical blood loss, cancer, chemotherapy, anemia associated with drug therapy for AIDS or hepatitis C virus, myelodysplastic disease, and anemia of chronic disease, especially when associated with rheumatoid arthritis or inflammatory bowel disease [12].

Anemia of chronic kidney disease should be treated with erythropoietin replacement. Treatment of anemia in persons receiving peritoneal dialysis or hematolysis, the most common indication for recombinant human erythropoietin, clearly increases the concentration of hemoglobin and decreases the need for blood transfusions and is arguably the standard of care [51,52]. The major benefit in patients who have chronic kidney disease is a partial correction of the hemoglobin concentration to 110 to 120 g/L. Increases beyond this level do not seem to offer additional benefits and are associated with increased cardiovascular mortality [53,54].

Treatment of anemia in patients who have predialysis stage 3 or 4 chronic kidney disease also increases the hemoglobin concentration and reduces the need for red blood cell transfusions but has not shown clear evidence for a beneficial or adverse effect on the progression of chronic kidney disease, on the timing of initiation of dialysis, or on subsequent mortality [55–59].

One hundred seventy-two subjects who had a hemoglobin less than 130 g/L, diabetes with evidence of nephropathy, and a creatinine clearance greater than 30 mL/min were assigned randomly to receive either early and complete anemia correction to attain normal hemoglobin levels (target, 130–150 g/L) or partial anemia correction (target, 105–115 g/L). The primary end point was change from baseline in left ventricular mass index at 15 months. Secondary end points included left ventricular end-systolic and end-diastolic volumes, left ventricular ejection fraction, and fractional shortening. Renal function was assessed by estimating the glomerular filtration rate by using the Cockcroft-Gault and simplified four-variable Modification of Diet in Renal Disease formulae at each scheduled visit. A self-administered 36-Item Short-Form Health Survey questionnaire was assessed at baseline and study end. Early and complete anemia correction to a target hemoglobin level of 130 to 150 g/L did not result in a decrease in left ventricular mass index at 15 months compared with patients maintained at a lower target hemoglobin level of 105 to 115 g/L. There were no statistically significant differences in any of the secondary or other exploratory echocardiographic parameters between the two study groups. No difference in estimated glomerular filtration rate was observed between the two study groups. Quality of life, however, improved significantly in patients who had early and complete hemoglobin correction ($P = .04$). There was no difference in adverse events or annual cardiac event rate between groups [60].

Several conditions may result in an inadequate response to erythropoietin therapy, including coexisting iron, vitamin $B_{12,}$ or folic acid deficiency, acute or chronic infections, inflammatory diseases, chronic blood loss, hemoglobinopathies, multiple myeloma, malnutrition, hemolysis, malignancy, hyperparathyroidism, and hypogonadism. Failure to respond to erythropoietin should trigger an evaluation for these conditions.

Blood transfusion is a common therapeutic medical intervention that is effective and rapid and is particularly helpful in the case of severe anemia (hemoglobin < 80 g/L) or life-threatening anemia. This intervention has been associated with increased survival rates in anemic patients who have myocardial infarction, but it also has been associated with multiple complications, including multiorgan failure and increased mortality in critically ill patients. When possible, blood transfusion should be avoided in anemia of chronic kidney disease and in anemia of chronic disease because of the associated risks such as iron overload and sensitization to HLA antigens [41,61].

Summary

Anemia is common in persons who have diabetes and is associated with increased morbidity and mortality. Diabetic patients are subject to developing anemia from all of the causes common to the general population, including iron deficiency anemia and anemia of chronic disease. The most common association of anemia with diabetes is through the development of chronic kidney disease. Diabetes has become the most common comorbid condition of end-stage renal disease in the United States.

The observations that chronic kidney disease is more common in diabetic patients than in patients who have chronic kidney disease of other etiologies, that anemia may occur earlier in diabetic patients than in patients who have other types of chronic kidney disease, and that anemia in diabetic patients often is found without measurable renal impairment suggest that the diabetic population may have a predilection to the development of anemia.

Treatment of anemia in diabetic patients is based on findings that anemia can be deleterious per se, particularly in association with cardiovascular comorbidity. In addition, anemia is associated with a poorer prognosis in diabetes-associated comorbid conditions, particularly in chronic kidney disease and cardiovascular disease. Finally, targeted correction of anemia in diabetic patients has improved patients' quality of life.

References

[1] Tran KH, Udden MM, Taffer GE, et al. Erythropoietin regulation of hematopoiesis is preserved in healthy elderly people. Clin Res 1993;41:116A.
[2] Zauber NP, Zauber AG. Hematologic data of healthy very old people. JAMA 1987;257: 2181–4.
[3] Salive ME, Cornoni-Huntley J, Guralnik JM, et al. Anemia and hemoglobin levels in older persons: relationship with age, gender, and health status. J Am Geriatr Soc 1992;40:489–96.
[4] Hsu CY, McCulloch CE, Curhan GC. Epidemiology of anemia associated with chronic renal insufficiency among adults in the United States: results from the Third National Health and Nutrition Examination Survey (NHANES III). J Am Soc Nephrol 2002;13:504–10.
[5] Artz AS, Fergusson D, Drinka PJ, et al. Prevalence of anemia in skilled-nursing home residents. Archives of Gerontology & Geriatrics 2004;39:201–6.
[6] Thomas DR, Cepeda OA. Evaluation and management of anemia in older individuals. Aging Health 2006;2:303–12.
[7] Cash JM, Sears DA. The anemia of chronic disease: spectrum of associated diseases in a series of unselected hospitalized patients. Am J Med 1989;87:638–44.
[8] Ania BJ, Suman VJ, Fairbanks VF, et al. Incidence of anemia in older people: an epidemiologic study in a well defined population. J Am Geriatr Soc 1997;45:825–31.
[9] Weber JP, Walsh PC, Peters CA, et al. Effect of reversible androgen deprivation on hemoglobin and serum immunoreactive erythropoietin in men. Am J Hematol 1991;36:190–4.
[10] Ellegala DB, Alden TD, Couture DE, et al. Anemia, testosterone, and pituitary adenoma in men. J Neurosurg 2003;98:974–7.
[11] Bogdanos J, Karamanolakis D, Milathianakis C, et al. Combined androgen blockade-induced anemia in prostate cancer patients without bone involvement. Anticancer Res 2003;23:1757–62.
[12] Kamenetz Y, Beloosesky Y, Zelter C, et al. Relationship between routine hematological parameters, serum IL-3, IL-6 and erythropoietin and mild anemia and degree of function in the elderly. Aging (Milano) 1998;10:32–8.
[13] Dharmarajan TS, Norkus EP. Mild anemia and the risk of falls in older adults from nursing homes and the community. J Am Med Dir Assoc 2004;5(6):395–400.
[14] Dharmarajan TS, Avula S, Norkus EP. Anemia increases risk for falls in hospitalized older adults: an evaluation of falls in 362 hospitalized, ambulatory, long-term care, and community patients. J Am Med Dir Assoc 2006;7(5):287–93.

[15] Herndon JG, Helmick CG, Sattin RW, et al. Chronic medical conditions and risk of fall injury events at home in older adults. J Am Geriatr Soc 1997;45(6):739–43.

[16] Steinberg KE. Anemia and falls. J Am Geriatr Soc 2006;7(5):327.

[17] Di Fazio I, Franzoni S, Fisoni GB, et al. Predictive role of single disease and their combination on recovery of balance and gait in disabled elderly patients. J Am Med Dir Assoc 2006;7: 208–11.

[18] Chaves P, Ashar T, Guralnik JM, et al. Looking at the relationship between hemoglobin concentration and previous mobility difficulty in older women: should the criteria used to define anemia in older people be changed? J Am Geriatr Soc 2002;50:1257–64.

[19] Levin A, Singer J, Thompson CR, et al. Prevalent left ventricular hypertrophy in the predialysis population: identifying opportunities for intervention. Am J Kidney Dis 1996;27:347–54.

[20] Wu WC, Rathore SS, Wang Y, et al. Blood transfusion in elderly patients with acute myocardial infarction. N Engl J Med 2001;345:1230–6.

[21] Ezekowitz JA, McAlister FA, Armstrong PW. Anemia is common in heart failure and is associated with poor outcomes: insights from a cohort of 12 065 patients with new-onset heart failure. Circulation 2003;107:223–5.

[22] McClellan WM, Flanders WD, Langston RD, et al. Anemia and renal insufficiency are independent risk factors for death among patients with congestive heart failure admitted to community hospitals: a population-based study. J Am Soc Nephrol 2002;13:1928–36.

[23] Milward EA, Grayson DA, Creasey H, et al. Evidence for association of anaemia with vascular dementia. Neuroreport 1999;10:2377–81.

[24] Cella D. Factors influencing quality of life in cancer patients: anemia and fatigue. Semin Oncol 1998;25(3 suppl 7):43–6.

[25] Thomas DR. Anemia: it's all about quality of life. J Am Med Dir Assoc 2007;8(2):80–2.

[26] Ferrucci L, Guralnik JM, Bandinelli S, et al. Unexplained anaemia in older persons is characterised by low erythropoietin and low levels of pro-inflammatory markers. Br J Hematol 2007;136:849–55.

[27] Artz AS, Fergusson D, Drinka PJ, et al. Mechanisms of unexplained anemia in the nursing home. J Am Geriatr Soc 2004;52:423–7.

[28] Nemeth E, Rivera S, Gabayan V, et al. IL-6 mediates hypoferremia of inflammation by inducing the synthesis of the iron regulatory hormone hepcidin. J Clin Invest 2004;113:1271–6.

[29] Jelkmann W. Proinflammatory cytokines lowering erythropoietin production. J Interferon Cytokine Res 1998;18:555–9.

[30] Means RT Jr, Krantz SB. Inhibition of human erythroid colony-forming units by gamma interferon can be corrected by recombinant human erythropoietin. Blood 1991;78:2564–7.

[31] Kazmi WH, Kausz AT, Khan S, et al. Anemia: an early complication of chronic renal insufficiency. Am J Kidney Dis 2001;38:803–12.

[32] Nissenson AR, Collins AJ, Hurley J, et al. Opportunities for improving the care of patients with chronic renal insufficiency: current practice patterns. J Am Soc Nephrol 2001;12: 1713–20.

[33] Hsu CY, Bates DW, Kuperman GJ, et al. Relationship between hematocrit and renal function in men and women. Kidney Int 2001;59:725–31.

[34] US Renal Data System. USRDS 2004 annual data report. The National Institutes of Health, National Institute of Diabetes and Digestive and Kidney Diseases; Bethesda (MD), 2004.

[35] Ma JZ, Ebben J, Xia H, et al. Hematocrit level and associated mortality in hemodialysis patients. J Am Soc Nephrol 1999;10:610–9.

[36] Thomas MC, Tsalamandris C, MacIsaac RJ, et al. The epidemiology of hemoglobin levels in patients with type 2 diabetes. AmJ Kidney Dis 2006;48:537–45.

[37] Thomas MC, MacIsaac RJ, Tsalamandris C, et al. Anemia in patients with type 1 diabetes. J Clin Endocrinol Metab 2004;89:4359–63.

[38] Astor BC, Muntner P, Levin A, et al. Association of kidney function with anemia: the Third National Health and Nutrition Examination Survey (1988–1994). Arch Intern Med 2002; 162:1401–8.

[39] Thomas MC, MacIsaac RJ, Tsalamandris C, et al. Unrecognized anemia in patients with diabetes: a cross-sectional survey. Diabetes Care 2003;26:1164–9.

[40] Craig KJ, Williams JD, Riley SG, et al. Anemia and diabetes in the absence of nephropathy. Diabetes Care 2005;28:1118–23.

[41] Weiss G, Goodnough L, et al. Anemia of chronic disease. N Engl J Med 2005;352(10):1011–23.

[42] Thomas DR. Nutritional anemia in older persons. In: Morley JE, Thomas DR, editors. Geriatric nutrition. Boca Raton (FL): CRC Press, Taylor and Francis Group; 2007. p. 487–96.

[43] Thomas DR. Anemia in older persons. In: Pathy JMS, Sinclair AJ, Morley JE, editors. Principles and practice of geriatric medicine. West Sussex (England): John Wiley & Sons, Ltd.; 2006.

[44] Cunieti E, Chiari MM, Monti M, et al. Distortion of iron status indices by acute inflammation in older hospitalized patients. Arch Gerontol Geriatr 2004;39(1):35–42.

[45] National Kidney Foundation Kidney/Disease Outcomes Quality Imitative. Clinical practice guidelines for anemia of chronic kidney disease: update 2001. Am J Kidney Dis 2001;37: S182–238.

[46] Mast AE, Blinder MA, Gronowski AM, et al. Clinical utility of the soluble transferrin receptor and comparison with serum ferritin in several populations. Clin Chem 1998;44:45–51.

[47] Dharmarajan TS, Adiga GU, Norkus EP. Vitamin B12 deficiency. Recognizing subtle symptoms in older adults. Geriatrics 2003;58(3):30–4, 30–8.

[48] Thompson JA, Gilliland DG, Prchal JT, et al. Effect of recombinant human erythropoietin combined with granulocyte/macrophage colony-stimulating factor in the treatment of patients with myelodysplastic syndrome. Blood 2000;95:1175–9.

[49] Ludwig H, Fritz E, Kotzmann H, et al. Erythropoietin treatment of anemia associated with multiple myeloma. N Engl J Med 1990;322:1693–9.

[50] National Kidney Foundation Kidney/Disease Outcomes Quality Imitative. Clinical practice guidelines for anemia of chronic kidney disease: update 2000. Am J Kidney Dis 2001; 37(Suppl 1):S182–238.

[51] Beusterien KM, Nissenson AR, Port FK, et al. The effects of recombinant human erythropoietin on functional health and well-being in chronic dialysis patients. J Am Soc Nephrol 1996;7:763–73.

[52] Tangalos EG, Hoggard JG, Murray AM, et al. Treatment of kidney disease and anemia in elderly, long-term care residents. J Am Med Dir Assoc 2004;5:H1–6.

[53] Drueke TB, Locatelli F, Clyne N, et al. Normalization of hemoglobin level in patients with chronic kidney disease and anemia. N Engl J Med 2006;355(20):2071–84.

[54] Singh AK, Szczech L, Tang KL, et al. Correction of anemia with epoetin alfa in chronic kidney disease. N Engl J Med 2006;355(20):2085–98.

[55] Cody J, Daly C, Campbell M, et al. Recombinant human erythropoietin for chronic renal failure anaemia in pre-dialysis patients. Cochrane Database Syst Rev 2006;4.

[56] Agarwal AK. Practical approach to the diagnosis and treatment of anemia associated with CKD in elderly. J Am Med Dir Assoc 2006;7:S7–12.

[57] Robinson BE. Epidemiology of chronic kidney disease and anemia. J Am Med Dir Assoc 2006;7:S3–6.

[58] Morley JE, Kim MJ, Haren MT, et al. Frailty and the aging male. Aging Male 2005;8: 135–40.

[59] Morley JE, Perry HM 3rd, Miller DK. Something about frailty. J Gerontol A Biol Sci Med Sci 2002;57:M698–704.

[60] Ritz E, Laville M, Bilous RW, et al. Target level for hemoglobin correction in patients with diabetes and CKD: primary results of the anemia correction in diabetes (ACORD) study. Am J Kidney Dis 2007;49:194–207.

[61] Woodman R, Ferrucci L, Guralnik J. Anemia in older adults. Curr Opin Hematol 2005; 12(2):123–8.

**ELSEVIER
SAUNDERS**

CLINICS IN
GERIATRIC
MEDICINE

Clin Geriatr Med 24 (2008) 541–549

Oral Diabetic Medications and the Geriatric Patient

Alan B. Silverberg, MD, FACP, FACE[a],*,
Kenneth Patrick L. Ligaray, MD[b]

[a]*Division of Endocrinology, Department of Internal Medicine, Saint Louis University School
of Medicine, 1402 South Grand Boulevard, St. Louis, MO 63104, USA*
[b]*UAB Health Center Montgomery, University of Alabama School of Medicine,
4371 Narrow Lane Road, Suite 200, Montgomery, AL 36116, USA*

Approximately 7% of the United States population have diabetes mellitus, and the vast majority (90%–95%) have Type II diabetes [1]. Diabetes mellitus is an expensive, chronic, sometimes debilitating, disease. According to a recent study in *Diabetes Care* [2], Americans will spend $174 billion dollars annually on diabetes care. Twenty percent of health care dollars are spent for individuals diagnosed with diabetes mellitus [2]. The prevalence of diabetes mellitus increases with increasing age. Approximately 21% of people above the age of 60 in the United States have diabetes mellitus [3]. Clinical trials have provided evidence for the necessity of tight glycemic control to prevent microvascular and possibly macrovascular complications of diabetes [4–7].

How tight the glycemic control should be is not agreed upon by all the professional organizations in endocrinology and diabetes. For example, the American Association of Clinical Endocrinologists (AACE) recommends a hemoglobin A1c (HbA1c) of 6.5% or less [8]. The American Diabetes Association (ADA) recommends an HbA1c goal of 7% or less [9]. Similarly, the Canadian Diabetes Association (CDA) recommends individualized targets, but says that most patients should have an HbA1c of 7% or less [10]. Should these recommendations apply to all geriatric patients? The American Geriatric Society (AGS) recommends an HbA1c of 7% or less if the individual is healthy and has a good functional status, but 8% or less if the individual is frail and has a short life expectancy [11].

* Corresponding author.
E-mail address: silverab@slu.edu (A.B. Silverberg).

The ACCORD trial (Action to Control Cardiovascular Risk in Diabetes) is a National Institutes of Health (NIH)-sponsored study of adults, aged 40 to 79 years, who had Type II diabetes mellitus and a high risk of developing cardiovascular disease. Part of the trial was to determine whether tight glucose control (HbA1c of less than 6%) would decrease cardiovascular endpoints. It was recently reported that there were increased deaths in the intensively treated group (goal for the HbA1c less than 6%) compared with the less-intensive glucose control group (goal for the HbA1c 7–7.9%). The intensive treatment group had 257 deaths and the less-intensive treatment group had 203 deaths. To date an analysis of the study data has not been published, but the intensive glucose treatment arm of the study has been stopped (www.accordtrial.org).

Glucose control, fasting and postprandial glucoses, should be as low as feasible without causing significant adverse events such as hypoglycemia. Hypoglycemia in the elderly might lead to cardiac problems such as angina or myocardial infarctions, falls, fractures, and disability, and subsequent frailty. What are the current oral medications available for the management of diabetes mellitus in elderly individuals?

Sulfonylurea medications

Sulfonylureas are all generic medications, which makes them inexpensive drugs for the management of Type II diabetes mellitus. They are insulin secretagoges that in some cases have been available for use for decades. They are typically divided into two groups, first-generation and second-generation medications. The first-generation sulfonylureas are chlorpropamide, acetoheximide, tolbutamide, and tolazamide. The main difference within each group is duration of action. Chlorpropamide has the longest duration of action at more than 48 hours, and tolbutamide the shortest at 6 to 12 hours. The first-generation sulfonylureas differ from the second-generation drugs in protein binding and milligram dosage requirement. The first-generation medications have high protein binding, which can lead to drug interactions because of drug displacement. The second-generation sultonylureas are largely free of drug interactions because of low protein binding, and require lower milligram doses to be effective. The second-generation sulfonylureas are glipizide, glyburide, and glimepiride. They differ slightly in duration of action, with glipizide having the shortest duration of action at 12 to 18 hours and glimepiride at 24 hours. Because patients who have diabetes, especially geriatric patients, are more likely to be on multiple medications, then the second-generation sulfonylurea medications are typically going to be used. Metabolic clearance of all of these medications is through renal or liver mechanisms [3,7,12]. Therefore, any impairment in renal or liver function will prevent the use of this class of medications. A summary of these medications is in Box 1.

The primary risk of these medications is hypoglycemia. This may be a more significant problem in the geriatric population because of decreased

---

Box 1. Sulfonylurea medications

Drugs
First-generation
Acetohexamide (Dymelor) 500–750 mg once or divided
Chlorpropamide (Diabenese) 250–375 mg once
Tolazamide (Tolinase) 250–500 mg once or divided
Tolbutamide (Orinase) 1000–2000 mg divided
Second-generation
Glimepiride (Amaryl) 1–8 mg once
Glipizide (Glucotrol) 10–40 mg once, (Glucotrol) XL 5–20 mg
once or divided
Glyburide (Diabeta, Micronase) 5–20 mg divided, (Glynase)
3–12 mg once or divided

Common adverse effects
Hypoglycemia
Weight gain

Concerns in the geriatric diabetes mellitus patient
Severe hypoglycemia secondary to renal or liver insufficiency

---

renal function, poor or irregular caloric intake, frequency of medication administration, and duration of action of the medication chosen. Therefore, in the elderly it seems prudent to start with low doses and carefully titrate the dose upward, if needed, and to use a medication with a short duration of action. Another problem in the geriatric patient who has diabetes is the presence of insulin deficiency in the nonobese individuals. Insulin secretogogue medications may not be effective in these individuals.

Monotherapy with sulfonylurea medications usually decreases HbA1c by 1.5%. If these medications are added to another oral diabetic medication, the decrease in HBA1c is only 1%. The near maximum effective dose of the second generation sulfonylureas is 50% of the maximal allowable dose.

Meglintinides

Another class of oral diabetic medication that has a similar mechanism of action to sulfonylurea medications comprises the meglintinides. There are two medications in this class, repaglinide (Prandin) and neteglinide (Starlix). Neither of these medications is available in a generic form. Meglintinides are rapidly absorbed and cleared through hepatic mechanisms. The medications need to be administered 30 minutes before meals. Their primary effect is on postprandial glucose levels. HbA1c levels decrease by approximately 1% with these medications [3,12]. A summary of the two medications is in Box 2.

Box 2. Meglintinide medications

Nateglinide (Starlix)
  60–120 mg three times daily before meals
  Cost/30 day supply: $84.60

Repaglinide (Prandin)
  1–4 mg three times daily before meals
  Cost/30 day supply: $77.40
  Cleared primarily by hepatic metabolism

Common adverse effects
  Headache
  Weight gain
  Diarrhea
  Dizziness
  Hypoglycemia

Concerns in the geriatric diabetes mellitus patient
  Compliance
  Hypoglycemia

In geriatric patients these first two classes of oral hypoglycemic medications may cause hypoglycemia, which might lead to mental status changes, falls, fractures, and resulting disability. Therefore, they should be started with low doses and carefully titrated to the lowest effective doses. Another reason to be cautious with these medications is the renal insufficiency associated with aging. Most of these medications are cleared through renal mechanisms. A third reason these medications may not be a good choice for geriatric patients is the associated pancreatic insufficiency in the nonobese patients.

Incretin medications

The newest class of diabetic drugs are the incretins. Incretins are gastrointestinal hormones that are secreted in response to glucose load. There are two available medications in this group: sitagliptin (Januvia) and exenatide (Byetta). Sitagliptin is an orally administered medication that is a dipeptidyl peptidase IV (DDP-4) inhibitor. Exenatide (Byetta) is an injectable drug that is a GLP-1 agonist.

GLP-1 and GIP are incretins synthesized by the intestine. They augment glucose stimulated insulin secretion, inhibit glucagon secretion, delay gastric empting, and as a result decrease postprandial glucose and fasting glucose values [13]. DDP-4 degrades these incretins very rapidly. The DDP-4 inhibitors prevent the breakdown of the endogenous incretins, and therefore prolong their duration of action [13,14].

DDP IV inhibitors improve fasting and postprandial glucose levels by stimulating insulin secretion and inhibiting glucagons secretion. Sitagliptin is well-tolerated with few side effects. Sitagliptin is currently approved for use as monotherapy or combined with metformin, thiazolidinediones (TZDs), or sulfonylurea medications. Hemoglobin A1c reductions are approximately 1%. A second DPP IV inhibitor, vildagliptin (Galvus) is awaiting Food and Drug Administration (FDA) approval [13–15].

Both sitagliptin and vildagliptin are recommended at 100 mg daily, and are administered as a single oral dose in the morning or divided for twice a day ingestion. The dose is reduced if there is moderate renal insufficiency (50% reduction in dose) or severe renal insufficiency (75% reduction in dose). These drugs are attractive choices for geriatric patients because they have few side effects and no associated hypoglycemia or weight loss; however, they are very expensive and may present a significant burden for individuals on limited incomes with or without a pharmacy benefit plan. In addition, there are no long-term outcome studies in patients who have diabetes, regardless of age.

Exenatide (Byetta) is the first available incretin mimetic. It is a 39-amino acid peptide isolated from the salivary secretions of *Heloderma suspectum* [16,17]. Like the incretin glucagon-like peptide-1, exenatide enhances glucose-dependent insulin secretion, decreases glucagon secretion, delays gastric emptying, promotes satiety, and at least in animal studies, preserves beta cell function [18]. Use of exenatide offers improvement of glycemic control and weight loss [19,20]; however, because weight loss may have detrimental effects in the geriatric population, experts recommended not using this drug until more data become available.

Alpha glucosidase inhibitors

Alpha glucosidase inhibitors work in the gastrointestinal tract to delay carbohydrate absorption and also increase GLP-1 levels [14,21,22]. There are two available drugs in the United States: miglitol (Glyset) and acarbose (Precose). In one study acarbose has been shown to prevent the onset of diabetes in a high risk population [23]. Although these drugs are not generic, they are not as expensive as TZDs and DPP-IV inhibitors.

Both miglitol and acarbose are available in 25 mg, 50 mg, and 100 mg tablet sizes. The maximum dose is 100 mg three times a day. To be effective, alpha glucosidase inhibitors must be administered with the first bite of food. To avoid discontinuation of the medication because of the common gastrointestinal side effects (flatus, abdominal pain, abdominal cramps), it is important to initiate administration of these medications at very low doses. The authors recommend starting at 25 mg at the largest meal and increasing the dose by 25 mg every 4 weeks. If there are no significant gastrointestinal side effects at 25 mg three times a day, then the dose can be gradually increased to 50 mg three times a day over the next 3 months.

The primary effect of alpha glucosidase inhibitors is on postprandial glucose. A modest decrease in hemoglobin A1c of 0.5 to 1.0 % is seen with miglitol and acarbose. There is no associated hypoglycemia with these medications [3].

The possible problems with alpha glucosidase inhibitor use in geriatric patients are the necessity for precise administration of the medication with the first bite of food and the frequency of administration (three times a day). These drugs are not approved for creatinine levels above 2 mg/dL (there are no safety data for this population). Liver function tests should be monitored periodically, especially if the patient is on the highest recommended dose (100 mg three times of day). A summary of these medications is in Box 3.

Metformin

Metformin, the only biguanide, has been used for diabetes management for decades, but its mode of action is still not fully understood [24,25]. In the presence of insulin it is known to decrease gluconeogenesis and increase glycogenolysis [26–29]. Studies suggest that early metformin effects also involve the adipose tissue [30]. Although it is recommended as a mainstay in therapy in most people who have Type II diabetes mellitus [31], a few issues need to be considered when used in elderly patients. Metformin is associated with anorexia and weight loss [32], both of which ultimately lead to increased frailty [33–35]. Metformin is not recommended for use in patients over 80 years of age [36] and in patients whose creatinine clearance is less than 60 to 70 mL/minute [37]. The latter is worth noting because renal failure may be masked in the elderly by sarcopenia [14]. Metformin is also best avoided in patients who have hepatic dysfunction, unstable congestive heart

---

Box 3. Alpha glucosidase inhibitors

Acarbose (Precose)
Miglitol (Glyset)
Doses are 50–100 mg three times daily with first bite of food
Begin with low doses and increase slowly to avoid or minimize
   side effects; start with 25 mg once a day and increase every
   4 weeks to 25 mg three times daily.
No hypoglycemia
Common adverse effects
   Abdominal pain
   Diarrhea
Concerns in the geriatric diabetes mellitus patient
   Compliance
   Gastrointestinal side effects

failure, metabolic acidosis, dehydration, or alcoholism. It should be with-held in patients hospitalized with an acute illness, and those undergoing radiocontrast studies or surgery during which the patient is at increased risk for lactic acidosis [25]. Even if clinically significant responses are seen at doses of at least 1500 mg/day, initial and maintenance doses should be conservative in the elderly and should not be titrated to the maximum dose of 2550 mg/day [38].

Thiazolidinediones

TZDs, pioglitazone and rosiglitazone, are pharmacologic ligands for a nuclear receptor known as peroxisome proliferators-activated receptor γ (PPAR- γ) [25]. Activation of this receptor modifies transcription of various genes that regulate carbohydrate and lipid metabolism [19]. Adiponectin en-hances insulin activity, and TZDs are known to increase adiponectin levels [14]. They exert favorable effects on markers of endothelial dysfunction [39] and inflammation, and also have the potential to stabilize or improve beta cell function [40]. These medications are excellent as monotherapy in pa-tients above 80 years of age [36], and are effective when added to metformin and sulfonyurea [40], exenatide [20], or even to insulin [41,42]. Pioglitazone proved to significantly reduce the risk of recurrent stroke [43]. Adverse ef-fects include weight gain, edema, anemia, and peripheral fractures in women [44]. Controversy regarding cardiovascular safety has recently been a major issue, especially after results of a landmark meta-analysis were released. The study concluded that rosiglitazone was associated with a significant increase in the risk of myocardial infarction and with an increase in the risk of death from cardiovascular causes that had borderline significance [44]. A more recent study focused in the elderly concluded that TZD treatment, primarily with rosiglitazone, was associated with an increased risk of congestive heart failure, acute myocardial infarction, and mortality when compared with other combination oral hypoglycemic agent treatments [45]. It cannot be denied, however, that major clinical trials support that TZDs have superior efficacy in improving and stabilizing glycemic control and have clinically meaningful vasculoprotective effects [46]. The role of rosiglitazone in diabe-tes prevention was demonstrated in the DREAM (Diabetes REduction Assessment with ramipril and rosiglitazone Medication) trial [47]. In light of recent cardiovascular safety concerns, good judgment should be employed and the use of TZDs should be individualized until further long-term data become available [48].

References

[1] Qaseem A, Vijan S, Snow V, et al. Glycemic control and type 2 diabetes mellitus. The optimal hemoglobin A1c targets. A guidance statement from the American College of Physicians. Ann Intern Med 2007;147(6):417–22.

[2] American Diabetes Association. Economic costs of diabetes in the US in 2007. Diabetes Care 2008;31(3):596–615.

[3] Rizvi A. Management of diabetes in older adults. Am J Med Sci 2007;333(1):35–47.

[4] UK Prospective Diabetes Study (UKPDS) Group. Intensive blood glucose control with sulfonylureas or insulin compared with conventional treatment and risk of complications in patients with type 2 diabetes (UKPDS 33). Lancet 1998;352:837–53.

[5] The Diabetes Control and Complication Trial Research Group. The Effect of intensive treatment of diabetes on the development and progression of long-term complications in insulin-dependent diabetes mellitus. N Engl J Med 1993;329:977–86.

[6] Diabetes Control and Complications Trial/Epidemioilogy of Diabetes Interventions and Complications (DCCT/EDIC) Study Research Group. Intensive diabetes treatment and cardiovascular disease in patients with type 1 diabetes. N Eng J Med 2005;353:2643–53.

[7] Bolen S, Feldman L, Vassy J, et al. Systematic review: comparative effectiveness and safety of oral medications for type 2 diabetes mellitus. Ann Intern Med 2007;147(6):386–99.

[8] Association of Clinical Endocrinologists. The American Association of Clinical Endocrinologists medical guidelines for the management of diabetes mellitus: the AACE system of intensive diabetes self-management–2002. Update. Endocr Pract 2002;8:40–82.

[9] American Diabetes Association. Standards of medical care in diabetes–2006. Diabetes Care 2006;29(Suppl 1):S4–42.

[10] California Healthcare Foundation/American Geriatrics Society Panel on Improving Care for Elders with Diabetes. Guidelines for improving the care of the older person with diabetes mellitus. J Am Geriatr Soc 2003;51:S265–80.

[11] Canadian Diabetes Association Clnical Practice Guidelines Expert Committee. Canadian Diabetes Association 2003 clinical practice guidelines for the prevention and management of diabetes in Canada. Can J Diabetes 2003;27(Suppl 2):S1–152.

[12] Drugs for diabetes. Treat Guidel Med Lett 2002;1(1):1–6.

[13] Ahren B, Simonsson E, Larsson H, et al. Inhibiton of dipeptidyl peptidase IV improves metabolic control over a 4-week study period in type 2 diabetes. Diabetes Care 2002;25: 869–75.

[14] Mazza A, Morley J. Update on diabetes in the elderly and the application of current therapeutics. J Am Med Dir Assoc 2007;8:489–92.

[15] Nauck M, Meininger G, Sheng D, et al. Efficacy and safety of the dipeptidyl peptidase-4 inhibitor, sitagliptin, compared with the sulfonylurea, glipizide, in patients with type 2 diabetes inadequately controlled on metformin alone: a randomized, double-blind, non-inferiority trial. Diabetes Obes Metab 2007;9:194–205.

[16] Eng J, Kleinman WA, Singh L, et al. Isolation and characterization of exendin-4, an exendin-3 analogue, from *Heloderma suspectum* venom. Further evidence for an exendin receptor on dispersed acini from guinea pig pancreas. J Biol Chem 1992;267(11):7402–5.

[17] Nelson P, Poon T, Guan X, et al. The incretin mimetic exenatide as a monotherapy in patients with type 2 diabetes. Diabetes Technol Ther 2007;9(4):317–26.

[18] Drucker DJ, Nauck MA. The incretin system: glucagon-like peptide-1 receptor agonists and dipeptidyl peptidase-4 inhibitors in type 2 diabetes. Lancet 2006;368(9548):1696–705.

[19] Mudaliar S, Henry RR. New oral therapies for type 2 diabetes mellitus: the glitazones or insulin sensitizers. Annu Rev Med 2001;52:239–57.

[20] Zinman B, Hoogwerf BJ, Durán García S, et al. The effect of adding exenatide to a thiazolidinedione in suboptimally controlled type 2 diabetes: a randomized trial. Ann Intern Med 2007;146(7):477–85.

[21] Lee A, Patrick P, Wishart J, et al. The effects of miglitol on glucagons-like peptide-1 secretion and appetite sensations in obese type 2 diabetics. Diabetes Obes Metab 2002;4:329–35.

[22] Deleon M, Chandurkar V, Albert S, et al. Glucagon-like peptide-1 response to acarbose in elderly type 2 diabetic subjects. Diabetes Res Clin Pract 2002;56:101–6.

[23] Chaisson JL, Josse RG, Gomis R, et al. Acarbose for prevention of type 2 diabetes mellitus: the STOP-NIDDM rendomised trial. Lancet 2002;359:2072–7.

[24] Bailey CJ, Turner RC. Metformin. N Engl J Med 1996;334:574-9.

[25] AACE Diabetes Mellitus Clinical Practice Guidelines Task Force. American Association of Clinical Endocrinologists medical guidelines for clinical practice for the management of diabetes mellitus. Endocr Pract 2007;13(Suppl 1):1-68.

[26] Inzucchi SE, Maggs DG, Spollett GR, et al. Efficacy and metabolic effects of metformin and troglitazone in type II diabetes mellitus. N Engl J Med 1998;338:867-72.

[27] Hundal RS, Krssak M, Dufour S, et al. Mechanism by which metformin reduces glucose production in type 2 diabetes. Diabetes 2000;49:2063-9.

[28] Wilcock C, Bailey CJ. Sites of metformin-stimulated glucose metabolism. Biochem Pharmacol 1990;39:1831-4.

[29] Stumvoll M, Nurjhan N, Perriello G, et al. Metabolic effects of metformin on non-insulin-dependent diabetes mellitus. N Engl J Med 1995;333:550-4.

[30] Eriksson A, Attvall S, Bonnier M, et al. Short-term effects of metformin in type 2 diabetes. Diabetes Obes Metab 2007;9(4):483-9.

[31] American Diabetes Association. Standards of medical care in diabetes–2007. Diabetes Care 2007;30:S4-41.

[32] Lee A, Morley JE. Metformin decreases food consumption and induces weight loss in subjects with obesity with type II non–insulin-dependent diabetes. Obes Res 1998;6:47-53.

[33] Morley JE, Kim MJ, Haren MT, et al. Frailty and the aging male [review]. Aging Male 2005; 8(3-4):135-40.

[34] Chapman IM. The anorexia of aging. Clin Geriatr Med 2007;23(4):735-56.

[35] Morley JE. Weight loss in the nursing home. J Am Med Dir Assoc 2007;8:201-4.

[36] Kim MJ, Rolland Y, Cepeda O, et al. Diabetes mellitus in older men. Aging Male 2006;9: 139-47.

[37] DeFronzo RA. Pharmacologic therapy for type 2 diabetes mellitus. Ann Intern Med 1999; 131:281-303.

[38] Metformin: drug information. Available at: www.uptodate.com. Accessed December 27, 2007.

[39] Albertini JP, McMorn SO, Chen H, et al. Effect of rosiglitazone on factors related to endothelial dysfunction in patients with type 2 diabetes mellitus. Atherosclerosis 2007;195(1): e159-66.

[40] Bell DS. Triple oral therapy for type 2 diabetes. Diabetes Res Clin Pract 2007;78(3):313-5.

[41] Berhanu P, Perez A, Yu S. Effect of pioglitazone in combination with insulin therapy on glycaemic control, insulin dose requirement and lipid profile in patients with type 2 diabetes previously poorly controlled with combination therapy. Diabetes Obes Metab 2007;9(4): 512-20.

[42] Hollander P, Yu D, Chou HS. Low-dose rosiglitazone in patients with insulin-requiring type 2 diabetes. Arch Intern Med 2007;167(12):1284-90.

[43] Wilcox R, Bousser MG, Betteridge DJ, et al. Effects of pioglitazone in patients with type 2 diabetes with or without previous stroke: results from PROACTIVE (PROspective pioglit Azone Clinical Trial In macroVascular Events) 04. Stroke 2007;38(3):865-73.

[44] Nissen SE, Wolski K. Effect of rosiglitazone on the risk of myocardial infarction and death from cardiovascular causes. N Engl J Med 2007;356(24):2457-71.

[45] Lipscombe LL, Gomes T, Lévesque LE, et al. Thiazolidinediones and cardiovascular outcomes in older patients with diabetes. JAMA 2007;298(22):2634-43.

[46] Goldberg RB. The new clinical trials with thiazolidinediones—DREAM, ADOPT, and CHICAGO: promises fulfilled? Curr Opin Lipidol 2007;18(4):435-42.

[47] DREAM (Diabetes REduction Assessment with ramipril and rosiglitazone Medication) Trial Investigators. Effect of rosiglitazone on the frequency of diabetes in patients with impaired glucose tolerance or impaired fasting glucose: a randomised controlled trial. Lancet 2006;368(9541):1096-105.

[48] Deeks ED, Keam SJ. Rosiglitazone: a review of its use in type 2 diabetes mellitus. Drugs 2007;67(18):2747-79.

ELSEVIER
SAUNDERS

CLINICS IN
GERIATRIC
MEDICINE

Clin Geriatr Med 24 (2008) 551–567

Diabetic Foot Management in the Elderly

E. Sharon Plummer, RN, BC, GNP, Stewart G. Albert, MD*

Department of Internal Medicine, Division of Endocrinology, Saint Louis University School of Medicine, 1402 South Grand Boulevard, St. Louis, MO 63104, USA

The elderly who have diabetes are at risk for foot ulcers and amputations [1–6]. People who do not have diabetes may at some time step on a splinter, or develop a blister from breaking in shoes, but will not develop ulcers or require amputation. Not everyone who has diabetes will be at high risk for foot-related complications; however, the elderly who have peripheral neuropathy, foot deformities, or peripheral vascular disease will be at especially high risk for complications [4–6]. There is a progressive increase in high-risk characteristics, with an almost doubling of the risk for each decade of life over 40 years of age. At the age of 80, the prevalence rate of complications may be as high as 22% for peripheral arterial disease, 35% for peripheral neuropathy, and 45% for any lower extremity disease. This article reviews the foot problems caused by abnormal pathophysiology found in those who have diabetes, and suggests a multidisciplinary program for screening and education to prevent ulcerations and amputation, and for the management of diabetic foot ulcers when they do occur.

The problem

Six percent of hospital admissions in people who have diabetes are related to foot ulcers [5,6]. The annual risk for developing a foot ulcer is 2%, the prevalence is 5% to 10%, and the lifetime risk is 15% to 25%. These ulcers heal 60% to 80% of the time, but are associated with amputation in 14% to 24%, and death in 5% to 13% of cases. After an amputation there is a 25% incidence of contralateral amputations within 3 years [5,6].

---

* Corresponding author.
  E-mail address: albertsg@slu.edu (S.G. Albert).

0749-0690/08/$ - see front matter © 2008 Elsevier Inc. All rights reserved.
doi:10.1016/j.cger.2008.03.009   *geriatric.theclinics.com*

Because the underlying pathology associated with the diabetes is symmetric (whether it is caused by neuropathy or peripheral vascular disease), after an amputation there is increased stress placed on the remaining limb, with resultant further ulceration.

Pathophysiology

The precursors for foot ulcers are related to the associated chronic complications of diabetes [2,3,7–10]. That is, peripheral neuropathy or neuropathy plus foot deformity may account for 60% of ulcers. Neuropathy plus vascular disease may account for 20%, and vascular disease alone for 20%. People who do not have diabetes are also at risk for hammertoe, claw toe, bunions and calluses; however in those who have diabetes, these foot deformities may be accentuated because of limited joint mobility at the ankle, subtalar, and first metatarsal phalangeal joint associated with diabetic neuromuscular abnormalities. There may be abnormal distribution of pressure, with the highest pressures over the big toe or over the first metatarsal joint, associated with development of so-called "mal perforans" ulcers. Previous ulceration places the patient at high risk of recurrence. Although healed ulcer scars may be structurally strong, the edges of the scar are subjected to high sheer stress, causing recurrence of the ulcer at the scar site. People who have diabetes may have peripheral edema from cardiac or renal causes. Edema in the foot may cause excessive pressure on the foot within the shoe, resulting in lateral or superior foot ulcers. Edema in the anterior tibial region maybe associated with chronic venous stasis ulcers. The patient may also be at risk for foot trauma, associated with pressure from overly tight or constricting shoes or from walking barefoot. There may be difficulties with foot care such as cutting nails or calluses because of difficulty reaching the foot, seeing the nails, or limited joint mobility. All of these factors combined with even minor trauma may present as a precursor to the development of a diabetic foot ulcer [7–10].

Peripheral neuropathy

The major peripheral neuropathy in diabetes is a sensory symmetric polyneuropathy, with a denervation of the longest nerves of the feet with progression upward in a stocking distribution. The first issue for consideration is the risk of the insensate foot subjected to acute trauma [11]. The individual who has neuropathy may suffer penetrating injury of the soft tissues caused by a foreign body, and being unable to sense the pain or the foreign body, will continue to ambulate and deepen the wound. The clinical correlates are to avoid walking barefoot or in socks alone, to avoid unprotected exposure of the toes with sandals, and to monitor for foreign bodies in shoes. The second issue is chronic low-grade pressure associated repetitive trauma, 1 to 5 kg/cm^2 for multiple impacts. This may be caused by loss of autonomic protective responses in gait and foot positioning, which in turn leads to blisters, calluses, and plantar (mal perforans) ulcers. The clinical correlate here is to wear appropriately fitting shoes. The third issue is increased pressure caused by overly tight shoes, in turn causing relative tissue ischemia. This is usually associated with the pressure greatest at lateral aspect of the shoe, and caused by 1 to 5 pounds per square inch over a prolonged duration of 10 hours. These types of ulcers are found in the lateral aspects of the foot or at the tops of the toes, and invariably any ulcers in these locations are caused by pressure from the shoe itself. The clinical correlates are to avoid pointed-toe shoes and overly tight shoes, and potentially to change shoes in the middle of the day, the so called "5-hour shoe wear," because it is likely that a second pair of shoes will not have the exact same pressure distribution.

Peripheral vascular disease

Diabetes is also associated with accelerated atherosclerosis and peripheral arterial disease (PAD) [5–10]. Patients may have additive effects on the peripheral circulation caused by underlying hypertension, hypercholesterolemia, and cigarettes. People who have PAD may have symptoms of intermittent claudication with the level pain situated at the level of the arterial insufficiency. More severe ischemia maybe associated with nocturnal pain and progression to rest pain. The symptoms of nocturnal pain may be described as being relieved by dependency and taking a few steps, whereas nocturnal neuropathic pain may not be alleviated by these maneuvers.

Foot deformities

People who have peripheral neuropathy may have loss of normal motor tone with resultant limited joint mobility, and abnormal rigidity to joint flexion [12]. Muscular weakness of the intrinsic foot muscles may be associated with shortened heel cords and excessive pressure over the forefoot, tips of toes, or over the first metatarsal head. The most severe neuropathic changes are associated with Charcot osteoarthropathy [13]. In this situation there is severe insensitivity and hypervascularity of the foot, with microfractures, collapse of the bones in the foot, and loss of the normal anatomy. This change in foot anatomy results in a maldistribution of pressure with midfoot ulcers.

Studies on prevention of complications

The role of a screening program has been evaluated in a randomized trial within an academic general medicine practice health care team [14]. Systems were developed as reminders for the health care providers to monitor patients' foot care practices, to encourage patient education, and to physically examine the feet at each office visit. There were 191 subjects in the intervention group and 205 in the control group. Outcomes at 1 year demonstrated positive changes in physician documentation and significant improvements in finding foot-related lesions such as calluses, fungal infections, and preulcerative lesions.

Patient education has become the standard of care for all prospective trials, and so there are few randomized trials with nonintervention (ie, a noneducation control group). An early-randomized trial by Malone and colleagues [15] at a Veterans Administration hospital evaluated an educational program in patients who had diabetes and high-risk foot characteristics of preexisting ulcers, or amputations. The intervention was randomized to 1 hour of foot education class plus take-home instructions, compared with a control population with no education. Follow up at 1 year showed significant decreased rates of repeat ulcers (5%versus 15%, $P<.005$) and decreased number of amputations (4% versus 12%, $P<.03$).

Studies of shoes for diabetic foot care

The use of prescription shoes has been considered a mainstay for preventive foot care. Early studies may be considered suggestive of benefit, but as reviewed [16], have been limited in scientific design, either in number of participants or lack of randomization. Uccioli and colleagues [17], alternately assigned subjects who had previous foot ulcers to prescription shoes (n = 33) or controls (no specific shoe recommendation, n = 36). After follow-up of 1 year, ulcers relapsed in 27.3% of those with prescription shoes and in 58.3% of those who continued to wear their own shoes ($P = .02$). Busch and Chantelau [18] compared the responses in patients who had a known history of foot ulcer. Sixty of them were allowed to obtain prescription shoes, whereas 32 were "forced to wear" their normal foot wear because of refusal of reimbursement by their insurance company. Follow-up at 42 months showed ulcer recurrence in 15% of those in prescription shoes versus 59% in the comparison group ($P<.001$). Reiber and colleagues [19] performed a randomized controlled trial on the effect of therapeutic footwear on foot reulceration. Four hundred people who had diabetes mellitus and previous foot ulcer or foot infection were randomized to three pairs of therapeutic shoes and three pairs of cork insoles, or three pairs of therapeutic shoes and three pairs of polyurethane insoles, or their usual shoes, and were followed up for 2 years. Overall there were no significant differences among the three allocation groups, with approximately 20% rate of reulceration within the 2-year follow-up; however approximately half the incidence of ulcer recurrence may be ascribed to non–shoe-related complications: trauma, ischemia, paronychia, or difficulties in self care.

Practical management

Recommendations by professional organizations on screening to prevent diabetic foot ulcers have been reviewed [3,20], and an approach is summarized in Table 1. Those people who have diabetes, without sensory neuropathy, vascular disease, or deformities (risk category "no neuropathy") may be examined annually. They may be given recommendations for wearing appropriately fitted shoes, and instructions for nail and callus care. Those

Table 1
Follow-up for foot care in persons who have diabetes mellitus

Risk category	Foot care visits	Footwear	Consultants
No neuropathy	Every year with education		
Neuropathy	Every 6 months	Properly fitted shoes with pressure-absorbing insoles	Foot care nurse or podiatrist for skin and nail care Pedorthist
Neuropathy plus deformity	Every 3 months	Extra-wide or extra-deep shoes with custom-molded plastazote or composite insoles	As above
Neuropathy with previous ulcer or previous partial amputation	Every 1–3 months	As above with rigid or rocker bottom soles Ankle-foot orthotics	As above and podiatrist or orthopedist Physical therapist Orthotist
Neuropathy with Charcot osteoarthropathy	Every 1–3 months	As above with custom-molded shoe/boot with high tops	As above
Vascular disease	Every 1–3 months	Determined by level of neuropathy above	As above and vascular surgeon

people in risk category "neuropathy" alone should be seen at 6 month intervals, with recommendations to be evaluated by a pedorthist (professionals who fits, designs and modifies shoes and orthotics), or other personnel interested in appropriately fitting athletic shoes or off-the-shelf prescription shoes. The shoes should be wide at the toe box, and deep enough to accommodate pressure-reducing insoles. These patients may require assistance in skin, callus, and nail care by a foot care nurse or podiatrist, especially if there are also difficulties with vision, flexibility, or inability in reaching their own feet. Those in risk category "neuropathy plus deformity" will require consultation with a pedorthist for extra deep or extra wide shoes. They may require molded plastazote or composite insoles to help with the gait and reduce foot pressure. Those patients who have had previous ulcers or partial amputations will need consultation with a pedorthist to provide shoes with rigid or rocker bottom soles along with the above modifications. Physical therapists may assist the patients in balance, strengthening, and heel cord lengthening. Orthotists my design ankle foot orthotics to alleviate foot drop. Those patients who have Charcot osteoarthropathy may have foot collapse with severe deformity and maldistribution of foot pressure. They may require custom-molded high top shoes with modification to the soles, insoles, and custom orthotics. These patients may benefit by consultations with podiatrists or orthopedists specialized in Charcot foot reconstruction surgery. Those people who have vascular disease will have increased risk for each level of neuropathy and deformity described above. They should be treated with close follow-up by foot care professionals, modifications to their shoes, appropriate consultations as delineated for their degree of neuropathy and deformity, and evaluation by vascular surgery. All of the shoe modifications are recommended to prevent recurrence of ulcers, but shoes themselves are insufficient to heal an open ulcer, which requires greater degrees of unweighting over the ulcer bed, and is describe below.

Specific approaches to foot care in older patients who have diabetes

Even though the underlying pathophysiology of the diabetic foot may sometimes seem grim, many experts believe that with proper care and protection, feet can last a lifetime. Achievement of this goal requires a team approach. The patient and family members have the most responsibility for performing the daily tasks that focus on prevention of problems. A multidisciplinary team is responsible for the assessment and education of the patient and treatment of the foot problems when they occur. These team members at each site will depend upon the resources at the facility, and the interests of the professionals. The team may include the primary geriatric physician, endocrinologist, podiatrist, vascular and orthopedic surgeons, nurse, physical therapist, pedorthist, prosthetist, and social worker [5]. Each of these team members has a part in the care and prevention of foot problems that pose a risk for amputation.

Foot care screening

Prevention of ulcers starts with foot care screening for all patients who have diabetes Table 1 [1]. This entails a detailed history of foot care practices, and physical examination of the feet for abnormal pressure sites, deformities, fungal infections, and sensory and vascular examinations. The foot screening initial assessment has the goals of early recognition and prevention of minor injury to the foot, of identification of risk factors or current problems, and of stratification of care. The initial history will take into account not only foot-related problems, but will also evaluate the active diagnoses, medications, allergies, and social systems of tobacco use, levels of ambulation, educational level, and support systems. The review of systems will also include evaluation of the musculoskeletal, neurologic, vascular, ophthalmologic, and skin integument. The history should include routine foot wear and foot care practices, such as how the patient resolves routine care of nails or calluses, what knowledge the person has regarding foot hydration or lubrication, if the person walks barefoot, and what knowledge the person has regarding routine inspection for foot-related problems.

The foot examination will include assessment of the skin (texture, integrity, subcutaneous bruising), toenails (dystrophic or overgrown), calluses (on the plantar surfaces or between toes), signs of web space infections (fungal or tinea), ulcerations, skin bacterial infections (cellulitis), or infection within ulcers. The musculoskeletal system should be evaluated looking at gait and any fixed or rigid deformities that will cause abnormal pressure distribution. The neurologic component of the foot examination will include assessment of dorsiflexion and plantar flexion, strength and range of motion, and plantar sensation with the use of the Semmes-Weinstein monofilament test (10 g), which tests for loss of protective sensation [2,3]. Further office based screening may include evaluation of skin temperature with infrared thermography to evaluate either for peripheral vascular disease (low skin temperature), or for evidence of maldistribution of pressure (high skin temperature of one foot compared with the other).

PAD may be screened by examining the dorsalis pedis and posterior tibial pulses. Arterial insufficiency may present with physical signs of cold skin, absent pulses, atrophic shiny appearance of skin, loss of hair on feet and toes, blanching on elevation, delayed venous filling on dependency (normal <15, moderate 15–40, severe >40 seconds), dependent rubor and gangrene. Further vascular assessment may include nonnvasive Doppler ankle/brachial indices (ABIs) in which a report of a ratio greater than 1.30 with noncompressible ("lead pipe," with abnormal waveforms) may be seen in severe calcified vessels. An ABI between 0.91 and 1.30 with normal waveforms is considered normal. Ratios between 0.41 and 0.9 are considered mild to moderate ischemia, and ratios less than 0.40 are considered severe ischemia. In a situation in which the Doppler examination cannot be interpreted because of noncompressible waveforms, toe systolic pressure may be determined by plethysmography, in which critical ischemia is a pressure less than 40 mm Hg. Treatment of symptoms of PAD includes smoking cessation, and exercise such as walking to tolerance. Patients should be cautioned against warming their feet by soaking in hot water or using heating pads. Cilostazol has been shown to significantly improve exercise tolerance, whereas pentoxyphylline has not been shown to be better than placebo [21].

Adjustment of the patient's medications to limit those that may exacerbate the ischemic symptoms, such as decreasing the use of diuretics and beta blockers whereas the appropriate use of angiotensin-converting enzyme inhibitors and calcium channel blockers may be helpful. Having the subject sleep in a reverse Trendelenburg position (head up-feet down position) has helped in some situations. Vascular surgery consultation may be obtained, and the indications for surgical intervention may be disability from job or exercise, rest pain, nonhealing ulcers, or gangrene. The further medical management of PAD also entails treatment for the high risk for cardiovascular disease and has been reviewed recently [22].

Education and behavioral therapy

Patient education involves two key concepts: inspection and protection. The feet are to be examined daily by the patient, checking for areas of redness, swelling, increased warmth, or ulceration. A handheld mirror may be needed to inspect the feet if there is a loss of flexibility. For a person who has vision loss, the foot inspection can be performed using the hands, feeling for any rough, open, draining, or warm areas. Many patients who have diabetes are unable to reach their feet because of obesity or arthritis, so another person will be needed to inspect the feet and provide care. In addition, the feet of the diabetic patient should be inspected at every health care visit. The second most important concept is protecting the foot against minor injury. The common causes of injury to the foot are from improperly fitted shoes, problems with nail or callus care, or trauma from walking without protective footwear.

Basic assessment

Footwear

A minor injury to the foot can set in motion a series of events that ends in amputation [7–10]. A thorough history of foot habits will help to identify any practice that could produce injury to the foot. The most common cause of foot injuries are shoes that are not properly fitted (too loose or too tight). In addition to examining the shoes worn to the clinic, inquiry should be made about other shoes worn.

A fundamental part of prevention is to evaluate the footwear for the proper fit, the ability to protect the foot from trauma, and the effects of the footwear on balance. The shape of the shoes should match the shape of the patient's feet. The patient who has loss of protective sensation often wears overly tight shoes to feel the shoe fit. Patients may be given a visual representation of the effect of an overly tight-fitting shoe by drawing the outline of a foot while they stand barefooted on a blank piece of paper. Comparison of the drawing of the foot with the shape of the shoe may emphasize to a patient areas of stress on the foot caused by pressure from the shoe. The shoes should be evaluated for the length and depth of the of the toe box. Shoes should be about 3/8 to 1/2 inch beyond the longest toe/toenail when standing [23]. Many elderly patients have thick toenails or toe deformities that can result in pressure ulcers under the nail or on the top of the toes if the shoe does not have enough depth.

The routine footwear should be assessed for the ability to provide protection and shock absorption. Shoes should have a sole that provides both protection against sharp objects (either kicked or stepped on) and shock absorbtion during ambulation. The shoes should be assessed for foreign bodies, such as nails protruding from the soles or palpable stitching from the inseams. Elderly patients may have complaints of foot, knee, hip, and back pain related to thinning fat pads in the feet, arthritis, or obesity. These painful symptoms may limit ambulation and interfere with health. Shoes with shock absorbing soles, such as an athletic shoes with mesh and leather toe boxes, are the best ''off-the-shelf'' choice, and may help to alleviate some of these symptoms [23]. Swimming shoes may be appropriate for water activities to protect against injury rather than going barefooted. Some elderly patients may not readily accept these styles and will require education and reinforcement of behaviors [24].

Socks

In addition to properly fitted shoes, choosing well-fitted socks may help protect against pressure and friction and also absorb moisture. Any color of sock is appropriate unless the person is allergic to the dye in the sock. Blends of cotton and synthetic fiber appear to be preferable to cotton alone, in that the blended fiber has the ability to dry faster. When moisture is wicked away from the skin there is less friction.

Skin

The skin, as the first line of defense against trauma and infections, should be kept supple. Routine washing with a mild soap and then immediate lubrication are basic measures for combating dry skin. Patients should be advised to keep the spaces between their toes dry to prevent tinea pedis (athlete's foot infection). Patients who have the loss of protective sensation in their feet may not sense these superficial infections, and when unrecognized they may lead to maceration and ulceration. Tinea infections must be aggressively treated with topical antibiotics to avoid web space ulcerations.

Corns and calluses resulting from thinning fat pads, bony prominences, and poorly fitted shoes may be precursors to ulceration. These hardened areas of skin, when accompanied by a loss of protective sensation, are not painful, may act as foreign bodies, and may lead to ulceration, especially if the callus/corn becomes bruised underneath. Treatment starts with reducing pressure and friction over the site by making changes in footwear described in the section on shoes. After the callus is thinned in the clinic with a scalpel or file, the patient or family can be taught to gently file the site weekly with an emery board to keep the callus thin and flexible.

Thick, hard, and misshapen toenails may also require foot care by a professional [25]. The patients may not have the tools, hand strength, or aptitude to cut their nails. Family members are often reluctant to provide care for fear of causing injury. A solution is for a professional to debride the nails, with a file or clippers, down to an appropriate length and thickness and then delegate the ongoing care to the patient or family member. This ongoing care of weekly filing with an emery board (designed for acrylic nails) will reduce the risk of trauma or skin injury from the patient's use of clippers.

A common complaint of "ingrown toenail" may be symptomatic of pressure on the side of the great toenail caused by overly tight or improperly fitted shoes. The appropriate treatment is to change the shape of the shoe to match the shape of the foot and then let the nail grow out. Sometimes trimming back the corner or the nail or placing a wisp of cotton under the corner of the nail and then wearing a sandal temporarily can relieve the pain from the nail. As the nail grows out, the side of the cuticle can be massaged with lotion after bathing to keep the nail from growing into the skin again. Properly fitted shoes are required to prevent further occurrences. If there is any sign of infection, antibiotics and drainage may be needed. Sometimes surgical intervention on the nail is required.

Musculoskeletal/gait

Elderly people who have fixed or rigid toes or foot deformities may have abnormal gait and balance. Reports of tripping or falling should be evaluated in the physical examination. Loss of dorsiflexion strength in the foot (foot drop) can lead to toe or foot drag during ambulation. A polypropylene shell ankle-foot orthotic (AFO), a brace that covers part of the plantar surface of the foot and extends to the upper calf, may be worn during ambulation to keep the foot at a 90° angle and limit drag. Patients who are plantar-flexed from a tight Achilles tendon have increased pressure on the toe tips and metatarsal heads, and referral to physical therapy for Achilles stretching exercises may be helpful.

Foot care for advanced complications

The patients who have loss of protective sensation, foot deformities, or peripheral vascular disease should be informed about their risk factors, re-educated at each visit, and followed by foot care professionals Table 1. Shoes should be appropriately deep and wide to accommodate shock absorbing insoles or orthotics. The patients may require prescription off-the-shelf shoes, and if there are foot deformities, may require custom-molded composite insoles. In patients who have Charcot osteoarthropathy with foot collapse, close collaboration by the foot specialist with the pedorthists and orthotists will be required to match the needs of the patient for specialized shoes with orthotics, custom-molded, extra-deep shoes, or high-top shoes to support the ankles.

People who have insensate feet may be educated to compensate for the loss of sensations by self-monitoring their feet for signs of inflammation such as warmth and redness. There is the recent description of having the patient monitor the foot temperature with an infrared thermometer for the early detection of low-grade trauma in the prevention of future ulcer development [26].

Diabetic foot ulcer management

When faced with a diabetic foot ulcer, there is the immediate decision analysis of whether the ulcer is infected, and if the ulcer is infected, whether this is a limb-threatening versus non–limb-threatening lesion. Recommendations that follow, outlined in Fig. 1, are derived from a wound categorization algorithm by the Infectious Disease Society of America (Table 2) [27,28].

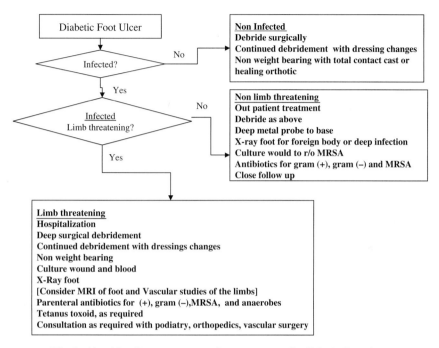

Fig. 1. Algorithm for assessment and management of a diabetic foot ulcer.

Table 2
Clinical classification of diabetic foot infections. Infectious Disease Society of America guidelines

Clinical manifestations of infections[a]	Infection severity
Wound lacking purulence or any manifestation of inflammation	Uninfected
Presence of two or more manifestations of inflammation (purulence or erythema, pain, tenderness, warmth or induration), but any cellulitis/erythema extend ≤2 cm around the ulcer, and infection is limited to the skin or superficial subcutaneous tissue; no other local complications or systemic illness	Mild
Infection (as above) in a patient who is systemically well and metabolically stable, but who has one or more of the following characteristics: cellulitis extending >2 cm, lymphangitic streaking, spread beneath the superficial fascia, deep-tissue abscess, gangrene and involvement of muscle, tendon, joint or bone	Moderate
Infection in a patient with systemic toxicity or metabolic instability (eg, fever, chills, tachycardia, hypotension, confusion, vomiting, leukocytosis, acidosis, severe hyperglycemia or azotemia)	Severe

[a] Foot ischemia may increase the severity of any infection and the presence of critical ischemia often makes the infection "Severe".

From Lipsky BA, Berendt AR, Deery HG, et al. Diagnosis and treatment of diabetic foot infections. Clin Infect Dis 2004;39:894.

The first decision is whether the ulcer is infected or noninfected. Initial assessment of the foot ulcer will evaluate for local and systemic signs of infection, and for the vascularity of limb. Assessment should include debridement of all necrotic tissue and eschar to viable tissue. Initial assessment should include the use of a blunt metal probe to delineate the extent and depth of the abscess or sinus tract drainage. Uninfected ulcers will usually have a clean base at presentation or after debridement (category "Uninfected," Table 2). Infected, but non–limb-threatening ulcers (category "Mild"), may have limited degrees of purulence, odor, necrosis, and clinical signs of inflammation, surrounding erythema 2 cm or less, and without localized increase in foot temperature. Localized lesions usually are not associated with systemic symptoms such as fever or acute deterioration in blood sugar. Infected limb-threatening lesions (category "Moderate") may be those with surrounding erythema greater than 2 cm beyond the ulcer bed, purulent, odorous, and localized increase in temperature (dermal thermometer $>2°$ difference between feet), a deep eschar, signs of tissue ischemia, or gangrene. The "probe to bone" test may be suggestive (87% sensitivity) of underlying osteomyelitis [29]. If there is a low pretest probability of osteomyelitis, the test is not found to have a high positive predictive value (57%). More importantly, a negative test in which the probe does not go deep to bone has a high specificity (91%) and high negative predictive value (98%) [29]. The patients in the "Severe" category of infection may have signs of systemic infection such as fever, sepsis, leukocytosis, or worsening of glycemic control. Vascularity of limb should be assessed by palpation of the dorsalis pedis and posterior tibial pulses, and by evaluation for signs of ischemia (blanching, rubor, loss of skin hair) and ankle/brachial indices if indicated, which may assist in prediction for wound healing.

Further diagnostic tests at this time may include radiographs of the foot. Plain films are of limited value but may demonstrate a foreign body, fractures, osteoarthropathy, gas in tissues, or osteomyelitis.

The decision sequence on the need for antibiotics in an open wound depends on the likelihood of localized or systemic infection. Those ulcers that are considered clinically uninfected do not require antibiotics, and may be treated with dressings and unweighting techniques as described below.

Those patients who have ulcers with localized signs of clinical infection that are non–limb-threatening after local debridement ("Mild" category) may be treated with oral antibiotics on an outpatient basis, with the ability of the patient to return for follow-up in 72 hours for clinical assessment [27,28]. The choice of antibiotics should provide coverage for gram-positive staphylococcus and streptococcus, and usually also gram-negative organisms. The recent prevalence of methacillin-resistant staphylococcus aureus (MRSA) in the outpatient setting has changed the empiric use of antibiotics [30,31] toward trimethoprim sulfamethoxazole, doxcycline, clindamycin, and levofloxacin rather than cephlexin, amoxicillin/clavulanate. The patients may be reassessed at weekly intervals for further debridement and re-evaluation of the type of dressings. Although the surface culture may not be indicative of deep-seeded infection, a culture taken at the initial assessment may help distinguish MRSA from methacillin-sensitive staphylococcus aureus (MSSA).

Wounds associated with limb-threatening or life-threatening infections (categories "Moderate" or "Severe") require hospitalization, parenteral antibiotics, vascular assessment, and surgical consultation. Parenteral antibiotics should provide broad-spectrum coverage for aerobic gram-positive and gram-negative organisms, anaerobic organisms, and coverage for MRSA. In-hospital management should include vancomycin, daptomycin, clindamycin, or linezolid for the MRSA, and coverage for gram-negative and anaerobic organisms (eg, imipenem/cilastatin, aztreonam and metronidazole, ampicillin/sulbactam, and fluoroquinolones supplemented with anaerobic coverage). The decisions on the urgency of surgical intervention should be made in concert with the surgical consultation regarding the severity of the illness and signs of sepsis or gangrene.

The wound should be assessed and surgically debrided down to the base [27,28]. Wounds are unable to adequately heal under an eschar. Debridement should be use of "sharp steel" to the base, or the level of bleeding of healthy tissues. The ulcer should be "wider than deep," which will allow wound packing for dressing changes. Chemical debridement with enzymes may help to loosen eschars but will not supplant surgical debridement. The major benefits of enzymes are to loosen necrotic debris over ulcer in ischemic areas.

The MRI of the foot has become the standard for evaluation for the diagnosis of osteomyelitis. It has supplanted other diagnostic tests such as technetium bone scans, which are nonspecific, and indium white blood cell (WBC) scans, which though more specific than technetium scans are more expensive and difficult to perform. The MRI, however, cannot distinguish changes of Charcot osteoarthropathy from osteomyelitis. The Charcot foot will also have clinical signs of warmth and redness caused by presumed new microfractures and hypervascularity of the limb. The differential diagnosis between osteomyelitis and Charcot osteoarthropathy will require other findings. Patients who have osteomyelitis may have systemic fever, blood glucose deterioration, elevated white blood cell counts, and clinical localization of an ulcer opening or fistula tract directly below the bony changes described on the MRI. The decision to use these imaging tests depends upon the clinical immediacy to find an osteomyelitis early. Surgery is immediately considered when there are signs of sepsis, fever, and limb ischemia. These imaging tests should not supplant open debridement of the ulcer to the wound base, with osteomyelitis more likely to be present if there is a deep-seated abscess. Alternatively, when the patient is clinically stable, there is the possibility to treat with antibiotics for 2 weeks and then repeat radiographs or diagnostic tests to evaluate for diagnostic signs of osteomyelitis.

Not all ulcers require amputation, not all osteomyelitis changes on nuclear medicine or MRI scans require immediate amputation. Osteomyelitis therapy is possible but difficult, and may require 1 to 2 weeks parenteral therapy followed by oral therapy for greater than 6 weeks, possibly up to 6 months. The decision for prolonged therapy depends on the functional level of the individual pre-amputation. That is, prolonged therapy may not be indicated to prevent partial toe or ray resections in which prolonged immobilization may adversely affect the lifestyle of the individual. Prolonged antibiotic therapy with careful monitoring may be indicated when the great toe, forefoot, or higher levels of amputation are the alternative. Those who have fixed osteomyelitis may not heal, and may develop a fissure tracking to the bone, and may then require surgical debridement of the sequestrum, the bone, or the limb. Consultation with surgery is indicated, especially when vascular reconstruction is considered. Amputation when necessary should be performed at the most distal site that will heal and that will allow appropriate prosthetics for later ambulation.

Wound dressing regimens will vary during the stages of the wound healing [32]. Initially the goal is debridement. Saline and Domboro (an acid media which is drying and has local effect on gram-negative pseudomonas overgrowth) with one of the numerous gauze dressings will help remove detritus. If there is a thick eschar, especially over an ischemic area, the eschar removal may be expedited with hydrocolloid dressings (DuoDERM, ConvaTec; Tegasorb, 3M Healthcare; Vigilon, Bard) which retain tissue factors. Enzymes collaginases (Accuzyme, Healthpoint; Santyl, Knoll/Smith & Nephew) may also loosen necrotic debris. During the follow-up, the wounds may become too moist, with maceration, and drying agents substituted (foam agents–Allevyn, [Smith & Nephew] Hydrasorb [Covidien], or alginates). Prolonged soaking or whirlpools are not recommended, as they may cause maceration and infections. "Antiseptics" agents that prevent regranulation such as Betadine, peroxide, and Dakins solution should be avoided.

Venous Stasis ulcers are associated with edema. Compression bandages (Coban, 3M Healthcare; Elastoplast, Beiersdorf-Jobst; Dome paste, Miles), Unna boots and multilayer systems (Profore, Smith & Nephew; Unna-Pak, Glenwood) are used with limb elevations.

Pressure reduction is critical for wound healing. Theoretically, this may be accomplished by non-weight bearing, use of bed rest, and wheelchairs. Practically, to allow the patient to resume activity, the standard therapy is a total contact cast [33]. This is a custom-molded, nonremovable cast, with closure over the toes to prevent trauma. The patient may also use crutches or a walker to further limit pressure on the limb. Some practitioners are uncomfortable with the closed cast, which limits the ability to monitor the ulcer bed for signs of infection. The cast also must be reapplied at 1- to 2-week intervals. Another alternative is the custom-molded neuropathic walker, ankle-foot healing orthotic. This is similar to the total contact cast, but it has a rigid bivalve removable outer boot, with a molded plastazote composite insole to limit and redistribute pressure at the ulcer surface. The advantage is that the patient and caregivers may monitor the course of the ulcer healing, and change dressings. The disadvantage is that the person may not wear the orthotic at all times, and may ambulate without the orthotic, or even barefoot. Other over-the-counter orthotics have been studied with similar rates of healing [34].

Adjuvant therapies are approved for nonhealing, noninfected ulcers after 3 to 6 weeks of optimal care. These therapies do not replace optimal care, should be reserved for specialized situations, and are possibly indicated in 10% to 15% of referrals. All of these adjuvant therapy trials demonstrated statistical improvement in wound healing compared with "standard care," which was usually a healing sandal, gauze, and saline dressing, rather than optimal care with healing orthotics and advanced dressings. Becaplermin (Regranex-recombinant human platelet derived growth factor) is applied to the wound bed, and may expedite the healing process [35]. Tissue-engineered skin, Apligraft (bilayer human dermal keratocytes, and epidermal fibroblasts in a bovine type 1 collagen lattice, Organogenesis/Novartis) [36] and Dermagraft (fetal fibroblasts, Advanced Tissue Sciences/Smith & Nephew) [37] are living-dermal equivalents. They may increase wound-healing rates. They are expensive and complicated in use, and should be limited to specialized centers. In a randomized trial, hyperbaric oxygen therapy, when added to standard therapy for patients who had nonhealing ulcers of 3 months duration, increased the early healing rate at 2 weeks but not after 4 weeks [38]. Specialized centers are exploring negative wound pressure (Wound Vac, KCI's V.A.C.) dressings [39]. Randomized studies for prophylactic Achilles tendon lengthening for plantar ulcers have demonstrated lower rates of ulcer recurrence, but possible poorer quality of life associated with the patient's inability to generate plantar torque after the surgery [40,41].

In summary, guidelines for diabetes foot care are available [1] and should be part of the routine care and evaluation of all patients. Those individuals who have good sensation, good vascularity, who have no deformities, and who are capable of reaching and seeing their feet may do well with education and reasonable approaches to footwear and foot care. Those who have advance diabetic complications of neuropathy or vascular insufficiency should be seen by professionals and given intensive education. An experienced team familiar with the progression of illness should follow those who have ulcers. The foot care team at each site will depend upon the resources at the facility, and the interests of the professionals (geriatrician, diabetologist, foot care specialist, orthopedic surgeon, orthotist, pedorthist, physical therapist, podiatrist, social service, and vascular surgeon). Not all ulcers or infections will require amputation.

References

[1] American Diabetes Association. Position statement. Standards of medical care in diabetes—2008. Diabetes Care 2008;31:S12–54.
[2] Boulton AJM, Kirsner RS, Vileikyte L. Neuropathic foot ulcers. N Engl J Med 2004;351: 48–55.

[3] Singh N, Armstrong DG, Lipsky BA. Preventing foot ulcers in patients with diabetes. JAMA 2005;293:217–28.

[4] Gregg EW, Sorlie P, Paulose-Ram R, et al. Prevalence of lower-extremity disease in the U.S. adult population ≥ 40 years of age with and without diabetes: 1999–2000 National Health and Nutrition Examination Survey. Diabetes Care 2004;27:1591–7.

[5] Levin ME. Pathogenesis and general management of foot lesions in the diabetic patient. In: Bowker JH, Pfeifer MA, editors. The diabetic foot. 6th edition. St. Louis (MO): Mosby; 2001. p. 219–60.

[6] Reiber GE. Epidemiology of foot ulcers and amputation in the diabetic foot. In: Bowker JH, Pfeifer MA, editors. The diabetic foot. 6th edition. St. Louis (MO): Mosby; 2001. p. 13–32.

[7] Pecoraro RE, Reiber GE, Burgess EM. Pathways to diabetic limb amputation: basis for prevention. Diabetes Care 1990;13:513–21.

[8] Boyko EJ, Ahroni JH, Cohen V, et al. Prediction of diabetic foot ulcer occurrence using commonly available clinical information: the Seattle Diabetic Foot Study. Diabetes Care 2006; 29:1202–7.

[9] Lavery LA, Armstrong DG, Wunderlich RP, et al. Risk factors for foot infections in individuals with diabetes. Diabetes Care 2006;29:1288–93.

[10] Reiber GE, Vileikyte L, Boyko EJ, et al. Causal pathways for incident lower-extremity ulcers in patients with diabetes from two settings. Diabetes Care 1999;22:157–62.

[11] Cavanagh PR, Ulbrecht JS, Caputo GM. The biomechanics of the foot in diabetes mellitus. In: Bowker JH, Pfeifer MA, editors. The diabetic foot. 6th edition. St. Louis (MO): Mosby; 2001. p. 125–96.

[12] Zimny S, Schatz H, Pfohl M. The role of limited joint mobility in diabetic patients with an at-risk foot. Diabetes Care 2004;27:942–6.

[13] Sanders LJ, Frykberg RG. Charcot neuropathy of the foot. In: Bowker JH, Pfeifer MA, editors. The diabetic foot. 6th edition. St. Louis (MO): Mosby; 2001. p. 439–66.

[14] Litzelman DK, Slemenda CW, Langefeld CD, et al. Reduction of lower extremity clinical abnormalities in patients with non–insulin-dependent diabetes mellitus. A randomized, controlled trial. Ann Intern Med 1993;19:36–41.

[15] Malone JM, Snyder M, Anderson G, et al. Prevention of amputation by diabetic education. Am J Surg 1989;58:520–3.

[16] Maciejewski ML, Reiber GE, Smith DG, et al. Effectiveness of diabetic therapeutic footwear in preventing reulceration. Diabetes Care 2004;27:1774–82.

[17] Uccioli L, Faglia E, Monticone G, et al. Manufactured shoes in the prevention of diabetic foot ulcers. Diabetes Care 1995;18:1376–8.

[18] Busch K, Chantelau E. Effectiveness of a new brand of stock "diabetic" shoes to protect against diabetic foot ulcer relapse: a prospective cohort study. Diabet Med 2003;20:665–9.

[19] Reiber GE, Smith DG, Wallace C, et al. Effect of therapeutic footwear on foot ulceration in patients with diabetes. A randomized controlled trial. JAMA 2002;287:2552–8.

[20] International consensus on the diabetic foot: practical guidelines [book on CD-ROM]. Noordwijkerhout, the Netherlands: International Working Group on the Diabetic Foot; 1999.

[21] American Diabetes Association. Position statement. Peripheral arterial disease in people with diabetes. Diabetes Care 2003;26:3333–41.

[22] Hankey GJ, Norman PE, Eikelboom JW. Medical treatment of peripheral arterial disease. JAMA 2006;295:547–53.

[23] Soulier SM, Godsey C, Asay ED, et al. The prevention of plantar ulceration in the diabetic foot through the use of running shoes. Diabetes Educ 1987;13:130–2.

[24] Plummer E. A comparison of foot care profiles in older and younger individual with end-stage renal disease. Masters thesis, Saint Louis University School of Nursing 1995.

[25] Janisse D. Pedorthic care of the diabetic foot. In: Bowker JH, Pfeifer MA, editors. The diabetic foot. 6th edition. St. Louis (MO): Mosby; 2001. p. 700–26.

[26] Lavery LA, Higgins KR, Lanctot DR, et al. Preventing diabetic foot ulcer recurrence in high-risk patients: use of temperature monitoring as a self-assessment tool. Diabetes Care 2007; 30:14–20.

[27] Rao N, Lipsky BA. Optimizing antimicrobial therapy in diabetic foot infections. Drugs 2007;67:195–214.

[28] Lipsky BA, Berendt AR, Deery HG, et al. Diagnosis and treatment of diabetic foot infections. Clin Infect Dis 2004;39:885–910.

[29] Lavery LA, Armstrong DG, Peters EJG, et al. Probe-to-bone test for diagnosing diabetic foot osteomyelitis: reliable or relic? Diabetes Care 2007;30:270–4.

[30] Moran GJ, Krishnadasan A, Gorwitz RJ, et al. Methicillin-resistant *S. aureus* infections among patients in the emergency department. N Engl J Med 2006;355:666–74.

[31] Klevens RM, Morrison MA, Nadle J, et al. Invasive methicillin-resistant *Staphylococcus aureus* infections in the United States. JAMA 2007;298:1763–71.

[32] Krasner DL, Sibbald RG. Diabetic foot ulcer care: assessment and management. In: Bowker JH, Pfeifer MA, editors. The diabetic foot. 6th edition. St. Louis (MO): Mosby; 2001. p. 283–300.

[33] Sinacore DR, Mueller M. Total-contact casting in the treatment of neuropathic ulcers. In: Bowker JH, Pfeifer MA, editors. The diabetic foot. 6th edition. St. Louis (MO): Mosby; 2001. p. 301–20.

[34] Piaggesi A, Macchiarini S, Rizzo L, et al. An off-the-shelf instant contact casting device for the management of diabetic foot ulcers: a randomized prospective trial versus traditional fiberglass cast. Diabetes Care 2007;30:586–90.

[35] Wieman TJ, Smiell JM, Su Y. Efficacy and safety of a topical gel formulation of recombinant human platelet-derived growth factor-BB (becaplermin) in patients with chronic neuropathic diabetic ulcers: a phase III randomized placebo-controlled double-blind study. Diabetes Care 1998;21:822–7.

[36] Veves A, Falanga V, Armstrong DG, et al. Graftskin, a human skin equivalent, is effective in the management of noninfected neuropathic diabetic foot ulcers: a prospective randomized multicenter clinical trial. Diabetes Care 2001;24:290–5.

[37] Marston WA, Hanft J, Norwood P, et al. The efficacy and safety of dermagraft in improving the healing of chronic diabetic foot ulcers: results of a prospective randomized trial. Diabetes Care 2003;26:1701–5.

[38] Kessler L, Bilbault P, Ortega F, et al. Hyperbaric oxygenation accelerates the healing rate of nonischemic chronic diabetic foot ulcers: a prospective randomized study. Diabetes Care 2003;26:2378–82.

[39] Lavery LA, Boulton AJ, Niezgoda JA, et al. A comparison of diabetic foot ulcer outcomes using negative pressure wound therapy versus historical standard of care. Int Wound J 2007; 4:103–13.

[40] Mueller MJ, Sinacore DR, Hastings MK, et al. Effect of Achilles tendon lengthening on neuropathic plantar ulcers: a randomized clinical trial. J Bone Joint Surg Am 2003;85A:1436–45.

[41] Mueller MJ, Sinacore DR, Hastings MK, et al. Impact of Achilles tendon lengthening on functional limitations and perceived disability in people with a neuropathic plantar ulcer. Diabetes Care 2004;27:1559–64.

**ELSEVIER
SAUNDERS**

Clin Geriatr Med 24 (2008) 569–572

CLINICS IN
GERIATRIC
MEDICINE

Index

Note: Page numbers of article titles are in **boldface** type.

0749-0690/08/$ - see front matter © 2008 Elsevier Inc. All rights reserved.
doi:10.1016/S0749-0690(08)00038-4

geriatric.theclinics.com